THE HEALING MYTH

THE HEALING MYTH
A Critique of the Modern Healing Movement

J. KEIR HOWARD

CASCADE *Books* • Eugene, Oregon

THE HEALING MYTH
A Critique of the Modern Healing Movement

Copyright © 2013 J. Keir Howard. All rights reserved. Except for brief quotations in critical publications or reviews, no part of this book may be reproduced in any manner without prior written permission from the publisher. Write: Permissions. Wipf and Stock Publishers, 199 W. 8th Ave., Suite 3, Eugene, OR 97401.

Cascade Books
An Imprint of Wipf and Stock Publishers
199 W. 8th Ave., Suite 3
Eugene, OR 97401

www.wipfandstock.com

ISBN 13: 978-1-62032-062-4

Cataloguing-in-Publication data:

Howard, J. Keir.

The healing myth : a critique of the modern healing movement / J. Keir Howard

x + 112 pp. ; 23 cm. Includes bibliographical references.

ISBN 13: 978-1-62032-062-4

1. Healing. 2. Spiritual healing. 3. Medicine—Religious aspects—Christianity. 4. Healing—Religious aspects. I. Title.

BT732.5 H69 2013

Manufactured in the U.S.A.

Contents

Preface | vii
Acknowledgments | ix

1 THE HEALING PHENOMENON | 1
2 BASIC APPROACHES: COMPLEMENTARY OR ALTERNATIVE? | 21
3 HEALING IN PRACTICE | 37
4 ASSESSING THE EVIDENCE | 51
5 INVESTIGATING FALSE CLAIMS | 65
6 CARING OR CURING? THE CHURCH'S MINISTRY | 91

Bibliography | 105

Preface

This book is concerned with the role of the Christian church in the care of the sick. There can be no doubting the fact that the church has seen it as part of its religious duty to provide care and comfort for the sick and needy from its earliest days. Recent years, however, have seen a significant change of emphasis from those early days, during which hospitals and hospices sprang up throughout Christendom as practical expressions of Christian charity. The consistent concern of those centers was on the care of the sick, provision for the poor and needy, and comfort for the dying. At the parish level, these were also the primary concerns of the clergy and their helpers. In more recent times, the modern missionary movement also built and staffed hospitals in which not only care, but also cure, were given equal importance—through the work of doctors, nurses, and other professional caregivers—alongside specifically religious activities. Christian charitable organizations continue these expressions of care and concern to the present. It was only in the late nineteenth century that the very different idea of a specific "ministry of healing" came to the fore, and with it a very different approach to the Christian duty of care for the sick. Religious healing through prayer and other means was now fostered, independent of the work of the medical professions. The emphasis on this form of ministry has blossomed, especially under the influence of the charismatic movement, until it has taken a central place in the life of many, if not most, churches.

The results of this change of emphasis from a ministry of care to a ministry of healing is the subject of this book. It will be argued that an honest and urgent appraisal of both current theory and current practice of what is called the church's healing ministry is needed. An honest recognition of the damage that this form of ministry has brought about in both individuals and congregations, particularly those associated with the

Preface

various schools of charismatic thought, is also necessary. Three issues are of particular concern, and will be addressed in the course of the book. In the first place, there needs to be a consistent understanding of what constitutes healing in any real sense. It is the basis of all that follows that the term "healing," as used in a medical context, and relating to sick people must include the reality of cure, measurable by the use of the proper criteria, otherwise the term becomes meaningless.

Secondly, the concept of miracle needs to be examined in relation to the claims of charismatic and other healers. In particular, it needs to be recognized that the term may not be used as some sort of "catch all" basket for anything not immediately understood or explicable. It will be argued, in fact, that miracle is a strictly religious term expressing an individual's subjective response to a personal deliverance.

Finally, there needs to be a proper validation of the claims made by modern healers. The Christian public, lay and ordained, continues to be inclined to take too much on trust, and to be remarkably naive in its attitude to the claims of the healing movement. It is rarely prepared to take the trouble to investigate these claims, which, if genuine, would be producing both remarkable and clearly observable effects on the levels of morbidity and mortality in society. The simple fact is that such effects are conspicuous by their absence.

It is the aim of this book, therefore, to redraw the boundaries for the church's ministry, and to raise the serious ethical and moral questions that have been very largely ignored by those in responsible positions in the Christian churches. These are issues that require to be addressed with urgency and objectivity by church leaders. By so doing, the church's proper role may be restored effectively by providing a framework in which both patient and family may come to terms with the inevitable reality of suffering and the inevitable and unavoidable reality of death rather than concentrating on misguided efforts to provide an imagined healing of illness. It is the provision of this necessary framework for proper care that the final part of this book will address.

It is hoped that this book will provide some counterbalance to the widespread confusion, misunderstanding, and extreme views that seem, all too often, to be the mark of what is called the church's healing ministry, as well as encouraging a more careful and critical consideration of the issues and a return to a proper role in the care of the sick.

J. Keir Howard
Ascension Day, 2012

Acknowledgments

My interest in the subject of this study goes back many years, and it would be impossible to mention all those friends, colleagues, and others who, by their conversations, debates, and their writings, have influenced my thinking about religious healing. My debt to them is enormous, even where I have disagreed with them, and I gratefully acknowledge their contributions to my own thought. Particular thanks, however, goes to my friend Professor Clyde Curry Smith, who reviewed a very early draft of the study with his usual incisiveness and critical eye for detail. Other friends have helped at different points along the road, and special thanks go to Nerys Parry and Tamar Posner, who have made comments, corrections, and criticisms at later stages in the book's period of gestation. Their expertise in the fields of psychology and psychotherapy has saved me from numerous solecisms and frank errors. I am also most grateful to my daughter Jacqueline Smith for going through the manuscript with a fine-tooth comb, drawing attention to infelicities in the text, as well as errors in grammar and syntax. Any remaining errors in the book are entirely my own. It is also a pleasure to record my grateful thanks to the editorial staff at Wipf and Stock, especially Dr. K. C. Hanson, editor in chief, and Christian Amundsen, assistant managing editor, who have carefully steered the book through to its completion with kindliness and courtesy at every stage. Finally, my thanks are due, as always, to my wife Dorothy for her ongoing support and encouragement, as well as having the grace to put up with me for fifty years!

1

The Healing Phenomenon

THE GROWTH OF INTEREST in, and practice of, what is referred to as "healing" in Christian circles in recent years has been remarkable. Venturing into this subject, however, is to wade into troubled and controversial waters, and there is no doubt that much of what follows will be controversial, and possibly even offensive to some. To start with, my use of the term "myth," to characterize the modern Christian healing movement, will no doubt cause a good many eyebrows to rise. Those sympathetic to the movement's aims and activities will no doubt consider the use of such a word both unnecessarily harsh and judgmental. It is, after all, a word that inevitably conjures up negative attitudes with regard to the matter under consideration.

The *Shorter Oxford English Dictionary* defines "myth" as, "a purely fictitious narrative usually involving supernatural persons, actions, or events, and embodying some popular idea concerning natural or historical phenomena." That will serve as a working definition, and it will be one of the aims of the present study to demonstrate that the great majority of the claims made by the advocates of religious healing may reasonably be characterized in this way. That some will be offended, and others angered, by such a judgment is a foregone conclusion; but at the same time it is hoped that there will also be those who will be prepared to give more careful and critical consideration to the issues that will be discussed in this study of what will be called religious healing, as a general term to cover the various forms of healing practice in Christian circles.

The Healing Myth

The starting point for this discussion is the widespread, and increasing public interest in, and acceptance and use of, the many varieties of alternative medicine to be found in the marketplace. The range is enormous from herbs to homeopathy, and among these forms of alternative medicine has to be placed the activities of those involved with religious healing in its various manifestations. Religious healing, by whatever name it may be presented, has taken a highly prominent position in today's Christian ministries, although, at the same time, it needs to be recognized that the movement as a whole is by no means homogenous, and a great many beliefs and practices, not all Christian by any means, hide under the umbrella of what is variously called "spiritual healing," "faith healing," "healing ministry," and what I have simply termed "religious healing." Such a wide variety of practices and beliefs would require a much larger and more detailed study than the one planned here were it to do justice to what is a very complex subject. Consequently, this short study is limited quite specifically to the role of the Christian church in the "healing" of disease and sickness, and particularly to an examination of the practices of those who advocate what has come to be called the "church's healing ministry." The brevity with which this complex matter is to be discussed may lead some to consider that I have not done adequate justice to either the beliefs or practices of the advocates of these forms of ministry. However, the primary concern will be to examine the evidence for and against the effectiveness of these various healing ministries. Can such ministrations be shown to have any curative effect on the pathological processes that cause disease and sickness, rather than providing no more than spiritual comfort and psychological support? Much has been claimed in support of healing ministries; the question that requires an answer is whether these claims are genuine or false.

It is unlikely that anyone would call it an exaggeration to state that, over the past forty or so years, the conviction that the Christian church should have a healing ministry has become virtually an article of faith across the great majority of communions. At the same time, it would also be true to observe that there has been remarkably little in the way of genuine critical examination and discussion within the Christian community as a whole, either of the claims made by the proponents of these healing ministries, or indeed of what exactly is meant by "healing." The term, indeed, is so slippery that it is almost impossible to establish a uniform and exact definition. The advocates of religious healing, whether clergy or lay, have, in fact, been highly articulate and very successful propagandists for their views and practices, with the result that "healing" (as noted above, a term almost always used without definition) has come to be accepted as a necessary ministry, virtually without question.

The Report of the Review Group set up by the bishops of the Church of England, published at the turn of this century, well sets out what has very largely become current thinking in most denominations of the Christian church. That document expresses the hope that, "this report will encourage all Anglicans to embrace what is sometimes called 'the full gospel'—that is the gospel preached with the hope of healing—so that it may become central to our mission."[1] In a similar vein, Roy Lawrence, an Anglican active in the healing movement, has written, "Christian Healing is a ministry for all who believe and profess themselves Christian and therefore for every local church . . . we must know beyond a doubt that a church which is not a healing church is hardly a church at all. So, every church a centre of healing? It is a necessity."[2]

Clearly the healing movement has arrived in a big way and is into a major "hard sell" advertising campaign. Doubts remain, however, both about the validity of its claims in general and, more especially, about its effectiveness with regard to the cure of genuine physical illness. In addition, the biblical foundation of much of its teaching requires serious scrutiny. These are matters that are open to serious question, but there seems to have been remarkably little in the way of critical examination from church leaders. As stated earlier, it is the purpose of this study to raise some of these critical questions and to encourage a greater level of critical thought among both ordained ministers and laypeople in the churches. Particular attention will be devoted to the claims of the healing movement to see whether they stand up to careful scrutiny, for at the end of the day the important question is simply, "Does it work?"

THE EARLY CHURCH BACKGROUND

I have argued elsewhere,[3] and on the basis of detailed critical exegesis, that, contrary to much popular Christian opinion, and the repeated assertions of the practitioners of religious healing, the New Testament as a whole displays remarkably little interest in the healing of sickness and nowhere suggests

1. Church of England Review Group, *A Time to Heal*, xviii.
2. Lawrence, "Every Church?" 84.
3. Howard, *Disease and Healing*; and Howard, *Medicine, Miracle and Myth*.

that it was a central and essential aspect of the proclamation of the gospel. There is certainly no suggestion within the New Testament documents that remarkable cures were happening on a daily basis in the early Christian communities, as is often suggested today. In fact, there is little foundation for assuming that the early Christian congregations undertook any form of extensive healing ministry. It was the story of the Good Samaritan that furnished the early Church with its model for the care of the sick and needy. As Ferngren puts it, "it was not curing but caring which constituted the chief ministry of the early Christian community to the sick";[4] and, unlike the pagan world, or even the Jewish community, the Christians extended their concern and care to all, irrespective of race or status.

Those who advocate a central place for a healing ministry, in the sense of curing disease, frequently tend to base their arguments on Mark 16:9–17. These verses form what is called the "longer" of the two main alternative endings of the Gospel, and paint a picture of the disciples being given what can only be described as magical powers to resist the venom of snakes and perform miracles. Unfortunately for those who wish to use these verses as proof-texts, they are universally recognized as secondary and constitute a second-century scribal addition to Mark, not forming part of the original Gospel. They represent a later attempt, and one that clearly pleased at least one scribe, to provide Mark with an ending that would bring it more into line with the other Gospels, with a set of post-resurrection appearances of Christ to his followers, but underpinned with the scribe's own or borrowed idiosyncratic theology.[5]

The New Testament, in fact, provides very little support for the burgeoning theologies of healing that have been developed in recent years. The emphasis of the first-century Christian communities was on caring for people in need and sickness, rather than on curing them. This is not the place to restate the arguments of my earlier studies in detail, although the main conclusions are worth setting out as a background to later considerations.

One thing should always be kept in mind when thinking about the diseases mentioned in the Bible. The understanding of the causes of different diseases and the pathological processes that gave rise to symptoms were lacking, even amongst the trained physicians of New Testament times. As a result, diseases tended to be classified simply on the basis of the symptoms or on the outward signs of the condition, as was the case, indeed, until very

---

4. Ferngren, "The Organisation of Care."
5. For details see Metzger, *Text*, 226–29.

recent times. As would be expected, therefore, the descriptions of disease in the New Testament are almost invariably symptomatic. Thus, the people who came to Jesus in the Gospels or to the apostles in the book of Acts are variously described as being paralyzed, lame, blind, and so forth. For the people of the time, the symptoms were the disease, as the underlying pathology remained unknown to them. Consequently, the various illnesses in which convulsions were the primary feature, for example, were simply lumped together, and no distinction would have been made between a disease such as genuine epilepsy on the one hand, and "hysterical" pseudo-convulsions on the other. It is unfortunate that this symptomatic approach also tends to be that of modern "healers" who, in general, have no real knowledge of the pathology and presentations of disease processes. Such a lack of understanding has, all too often, been a recipe for disaster, a matter that will be discussed later.

It has also to be remembered that the primary aims of the evangelists were theological, and thus the Gospel traditions have undergone progressive editorial adjustments to ensure that the evangelistic and teaching needs of the young communities were being met as they began to expand into the Roman world. These considerations mean that considerable care needs to be taken in interpreting the nature of the healing stories of Jesus and the apostles. Nonetheless, there are adequate clues in the Gospel narratives to be able to draw broad conclusions about these stories. These clues come in the form of the symptoms and signs that are described, coupled with the information about the healing methods that Jesus appears to have used, and together they provide support for the conclusion that the majority of the conditions treated came within the general category of what may be termed "functional" or psychosomatic. A high proportion seem to have been cases of what are called conversion disorders or somatoform disorders, those conditions that used to be called "hysterical neuroses." The term "conversion" in this context has nothing to do with religious conversion, but rather describes the situation when someone in a highly unpleasant and stressful situation escapes from it by converting the mental stress into physical symptoms of illness. Such conditions are common in all human societies, although cultural factors often affect the way in which they manifest themselves. An example of such a somatoform illness is seen in the case of the "possessed" man from Capernaum (Mark 1:21–28) in which psychological conflicts were transformed into bodily symptoms and complaints. In the discussion that follows, I shall use the term somatoform disorder to avoid any possibility of confusion with religious conversion.

What was true of the ministry of Jesus seems also to have been true of the illnesses treated by the apostles, although the Lukan witness of Acts probably may not be treated with the same degree of confidence as the Markan tradition of the ministry of Jesus. The pattern that emerges from a study of the diseases treated by Jesus, and probably also by the apostles, is thus one of conditions having their origin in those forms of mental disorder that closely mimic conditions that have a genuine physical pathology. Conditions of this nature tend to present as paralysis; lameness; loss of balance; dramatic convulsions; severe pain without pathology; and various sensory defects such as deafness, dumbness, and, more rarely, blindness. The physical symptoms closely mimic the features of genuine physical illness, but there is no evidence of the corresponding pathology of the physical disease itself. The condition is real, but the cause is psychosomatic rather than physical, and they form part of the spectrum of psychosocial disease and, in particular, the somatoform disorders. I have argued that there is a reasonable degree of certainty that it was diseases of this type that formed the most common, by far, of the conditions dealt with by Jesus and his apostles.

It also seems very possible that some of the examples of blindness recorded in the Gospels and Acts may have fallen into this category as well. However, in view of the way in which Jesus is recorded as healing the blind by the use of touch, it seems more likely that most, if not all, cases of blindness were likely to have been the result of severe cataracts (a condition that was very common in the eastern Mediterranean region, and remains common in areas of high natural exposure to ultra-violet light) treated by him with the use of the ancient method of manual couching. It is essentially a simple maneuver, performed by placing pressure on the eyeball causing over-ripe cataracts to fall back into the eye cavity (the posterior chamber) thus clearing the visual pathway. The clearest description occurs in Mark 8:22–26 (the blind man of Bethsaida) and I have discussed this in detail elsewhere.[6] It is a method still used by traditional healers in the Middle East and on the Indian subcontinent. In out of the way and isolated areas, the villagers will still wait eagerly for the arrival of the "eye man" to deal with cataracts by this method, especially among the elderly. There are very few other forms of genuine physical disorder mentioned in the Gospel narratives, other than such self-limiting conditions as febrile illnesses and diarrhea.

6. Howard, *Disease and Healing*, 106–12.

Mention should also be made of what most English versions of the Bible still refer to as "leprosy," a loose and general term in the biblical texts for various skin conditions, particularly psoriasis, and not the modern condition of Hansen's disease, which is caused by a specific organism related to the bacterium causing tuberculosis. It is extraordinary that this mistranslation has persisted for so long, since it has been recognized for well over a hundred years that the word "leprosy," "was ill-chosen in the first instance, and has continued to confuse the whole subject down to the present time."[7] A close reading of the Gospels would suggest that people with this condition were "declared clean" by Jesus, rather than being cured. The condition is mentioned only in the Synoptic Gospels, and it is of interest to note that the lack of feeling in the skin, which is the primary presenting symptom of Hansen's disease, is never mentioned in the Bible.

It needs to be emphasized, therefore, that descriptions of conditions which may, with some degree of confidence, be considered as true organic diseases, and occurring without a dominant functional or psychosomatic component, are very limited indeed in the Gospel stories. The historical record of the Gospels provides a consistent and entirely reasonable picture of Jesus as a prophetic healer of certain forms of illness: predominantly psychological, somatoform disorders, together with a smaller number of physical illnesses, for which the accepted means of folk medicine were appropriate and effective. The Gospel picture of Jesus as "healer" is both medically sound and completely convincing. Similarly, the accounts of healing in the book of Acts would indicate that the same broad conclusions apply to the work of the apostles. The very limited evidence from Acts would suggest that the work of the apostles followed very much the same pattern as that of Jesus, and, as in the Gospels, there is a predominance of what appear to be "psychosomatic" illnesses in these narratives.

The remarkably few stories of cures of physical disease arising from true organic pathology in the New Testament narratives need to be set against the claims of the modern healing movement. James D. G. Dunn has commented that it is "striking that no instances of healing purely physical injuries or mending broken limbs are attributed to Jesus in the earliest stratum of tradition—that is to say, there is no instance of a healing miracle which falls clearly outside the general category of psychosomatic illnesses."[8] To say "no instance" is a slight exaggeration in view of

7. Greenwood, "Leprosy," 76–78.
8. Dunn, *Jesus*, 71.

the evidence that suggests that Jesus used the techniques of folk medicine to deal with certain conditions such as cataracts, as noted above, but the broad truth of Dunn's statement cannot be denied. It is only in the later traditions, with their tendency to elaborate and expand as part of a program to defend and vindicate the gospel message, a tendency seen particularly in Luke–Acts, that stories are recounted in which both Jesus and the apostles are represented as dealing with larger numbers of physical and chronic disorders. The end result of this process is seen in the radical and exaggerated claims made for the followers of Jesus in the apocryphal second century, so-called "longer" ending, of Mark (16:9–20) discussed above, in which the disciples are purportedly given what are, to all intents and purposes, magical powers. It was observed earlier in this argument that the claims of the modern healing movement are based, to a very large extent, on this late textual emendation, a very shaky foundation for building a theology to say the least.

The extent of any healing ministry in the first-century Christian communities may be assessed only on the information in the New Testament letters. There are, in fact, very few references to healing outside the Gospels and Acts, although there is some suggestion from Paul's writings that some form of healing practice existed in the early community. It is clear, however, that he did not give it a high profile in his ministry, and the only references to "gifts of healing" occur at 1 Cor 12:9, 28, 30. In view of the complete absence of any other references to such gifts in the New Testament, it is difficult to see how these few verses can sustain the weight that has been placed upon them in support of healing gifts in today's Church. Furthermore, it also seems very possible that, whatever such gifts were, they were something unique to the Christians in Corinth, and it is, in fact, not by any means improbable that the healing to which Paul refers was something other than physical healing. It is, therefore, worth making a brief comment on what Paul actually had to say to the Corinthians on the subject of the "gifts of healing." He used the noun *iama* to denote healing, a word that usually means "a remedy," "a medicine," or "a method of curing." It is a rare word, occurring only in this passage in the New Testament, although the related verb is used both literally, particularly in Luke's Gospel, as well as metaphorically, for the restoration of people from all sorts of ills in other passages. In view of the fact that this noun is not found elsewhere in the New Testament, it may be wise to exercise caution before assuming automatically that the "gifts of healing" refer to the cure of physical disease. As

The Healing Phenomenon

I have remarked elsewhere, a "gift that enabled some to provide physical healing to other members of the congregation seems out of place in a list that related, in all other aspects, to the spiritual welfare and functioning of the community."[9] It would seem much more likely, in view of the context, to see these specific gifts being associated with the restoration of people to what might be termed spiritual health, perhaps when depressed, downhearted, and despondent. It is this type of situation that is also in view in the letter of James (5:14, 15), where the advice is given to call in the elders of the congregation to minister to those affected in such ways. Whatever the situation may have been, it is important to remember that the church in Corinth was probably the most disorderly and disordered of any of the communities that Paul or his companions had established, and it hardly represents a community that would provide an ideal for others to imitate. Care should be taken, therefore, in making any presumptions about using the practices of the Corinthians as a foundation for what Christians should be doing in later times.

The remainder of the New Testament gives even less foundation for assuming that there was any extensive healing ministry in the early Christian congregations, and there is certainly no evidence in any of the New Testament letters that physical diseases were ever healed by other than natural processes. Further, and very importantly, the New Testament letters make no reference to the practice of exorcism, nor indeed to the idea of demonic possession at all. There is nothing in the writings of Paul that would suggest that he was ever involved in such practices, nor do any of the other New Testament documents suggest that such practices were part of the normal activities of the early Christian community.

On the other hand, prayer for the sick formed an important ingredient in pastoral care, and this is made very clear in numerous places in the New Testament letters. However, the recognition that prayer for the sick was an important part of pastoral ministry is a very far cry from saying that there was an automatic assumption within the community that such prayer would result in the cure of the sick person. It is very clear that in some cases it did not, including that of Paul himself (2 Cor 12:7). It is important to bear in mind that Paul's letters are among the earliest documents in the New Testament. They predate Mark, which is generally regarded as the earliest Gospel, by at least ten years, and predate the other Gospels by substantially longer periods, in the case of John probably by

---

9. Howard, *Medicine, Miracle and Myth*, 92.

nearly half a century. It is significant, therefore, that so little attention is paid to the issue of healing in the Pauline or other letters. There is little, if anything, in any of the New Testament letters to suggest that "healing," as opposed to "caring," was considered an indispensable part of the evangelistic or pastoral activity of the early Christian communities.

Indeed, it is of importance to note that Paul himself seems to have made no attempt to heal his own colleagues when they were sick. One notes, for example, his remarks about Epaphroditus at Phil 2:25–30, as well as the references to Timothy (1 Tim 5:23) and Trophimus (2 Tim 4:20) in the Pastoral Epistles which, although unlikely to have come from Paul's hand, would certainly seem to embody genuine Pauline memories. The advice given to Timothy is, in fact, very far removed from any ideas of special or "miraculous" healing. The prescription comes straight out of the methods of Greek medical practice for dealing with people whose constitutions were not strong. Neither Paul, nor his colleagues, considered that Christian faith provided either immunity from disease or an assurance of its cure.

Similarly, there is little evidence that "healing" was a major issue in the writings of the Apostolic Fathers, such as the letters of Clement, Polycarp, and Ignatius in the late first and early second centuries. The letter of Ignatius to Polycarp, for example, inculcates care of the sick as part of Christian duty rather than a ministry of healing the sick, although the meaning of the phrase, "bear with all the sick" is not entirely clear.[10] It is not until the latter half of the second century and onwards that there is any emphasis on what might be termed a "healing ministry" as something different from the normal pastoral care of the sick. These later developments may well represent reactions to the work of heterodox sects, such as the Montanists (a sort of early equivalent of the charismatic movement) and, perhaps in particular, to the growth of pagan healing cults, particularly those associated with Asclepius. The Christian establishment wanted to show that its god was as powerful, or more powerful, than the gods of the pagans. There are references to the healing of the sick and casting out demons in the writings of Justin Martyr, Irenaeus, and Origen in the latter half of the second century, but even Origen, who claimed to have witnessed miracles, fails to provide a specific example,[11] and the same is true of Irenaeus,[12] who makes great claims for the true church, over against the heretics, but fails to provide a

---

10. Ignatius to Polycarp 1:3.
11. Origen, *Contra Celsum* 1:46; 2:8.
12. Irenaeus, *Adversus Haereses* 2.31.2—32.4.

single example. It is not until the third century that references become more common. Yet even the probably late third-century *Didascalia Apostolorum* (a manual to guide all aspects of Christian living) for example, utilizes the language of healing solely in relation to spiritual matters, and there is no suggestion anywhere of an anticipation that the cure of disease might be brought about by miraculous means. Furthermore, these later references to healing miracles are all couched in the conventional language of Christian apologetic, and they are remarkably short on concrete examples. When one considers the apologetic value of being able to cite specific examples to counter pagan claims, it is significant that not one Christian writer actually does so, suggesting that the best evidence was no more than hearsay or the turning of the New Testament stories into contemporary legends.

The emphasis in early Christianity was placed squarely on the care of the sick, and the terminology of healing was used largely in a metaphorical sense of the restoration of the sinner to spiritual health. These writings provide little evidence that the early Christian communities expected miraculous cures or anticipated that illness would do other than run its natural course. The emphasis was on sustaining and helping the sick in their situation by a practical ministry of caring and prayer. The fact of the matter seems to be, therefore, that the early church did not demonstrate any great interest in either miracle or religious healing practices until a much later stage of its development, from the late second century onwards. The modern healing movement, especially in its charismatic forms, cannot look to the New Testament or the early Church Fathers to provide a basis for its activities, but only to a much later stage of development when the Church was attempting to be competitive with paganism and apparently using the same methods.

The primary question that has to be asked, therefore, relates to the church's function in relation to illness. Is it to provide healing or is it to provide support and care for the sick? Is the mission of the church to attempt the cure of disease or is its ministry what has been historically understood as "the cure of souls"? In giving consideration to these matters, it has to be borne in mind that very few Christian ministers are medically qualified, and therefore competent, to assess the nature of a person's illness. As I have remarked elsewhere, "effective therapy is based on rational and adequate diagnosis, and it this absence of any proper diagnosis which makes nonsense of so much that passes for "healing" in the practice of healing ministries."[13] The question of the Church's function in respect of sickness is

13. Howard, *Disease and Healing*, 297.

one that requires urgent consideration, but it cannot be answered without a review of current practice and an examination of its results, and especially its dangers, dangers that apply particularly to the charismatic/pentecostal type of "healing" that has come to be the predominant manifestation of healing ministries in the Christian church today. Before examining the practices of healing, however, it is necessary to give some thought to the difficult issue of what is actually meant by the term "healing."

THE CONTEMPORARY CONTEXT OF "HEALING"

It is one of the paradoxes of life that it is easier to provide a definition of disease or ill health than it is of health or healing. The term "healing," in particular, is one that is frequently used very vaguely and without adequate definition, and this is nowhere more apparent than in the writings of those associated with the healing movement in the modern church, as well as other forms of alternative medicine. The growth of various healing practices in the church has been phenomenal, particularly over the past forty years or so, and has very largely grown in parallel with the charismatic movement, which itself places a major emphasis on "healing," as well as on other phenomena that it considers manifestations of God's Spirit, particularly what is called "the gift of tongues." This quite remarkable explosion of interest in and practice of religious healing, however, would seem to be, in some sense at least, little more than a "me too" response of the church, aligning itself with the growing trend throughout western society of the practice of "alternative medicine."

The term "alternative medicine" is not a particularly good one since, as an editorial in the *Journal of the American Medical Association* noted, "There is no alternative medicine. There is only scientifically proven, evidence-based medicine supported by solid data, or unproven medicine, for which scientific evidence is lacking."[14] The term, however, is here to stay and is generally used of the practice of various quasi-therapeutic methods in the place of normal, evidence-based medical practice. Homeopathy and the more arcane practices of iridology, reflexology, and so forth, may be set into this category. Good evidence for the effectiveness of these methods in the cure of disease, rather than the induction of "feel good" responses, is completely lacking in spite of the many studies that have been undertaken

---

14. Anonymous, "Editorial," 1618–19.

to investigate them. However, for as long as people believe that such practices actually work, there will always be a market for them.

The surprising aspect of this growth of unorthodox practice is that it has taken place against a background of the most significant advances in the treatment and cure of disease in human history. James Le Fanu has remarked that the "history of medicine in the fifty years since the end of the Second World War ranks as one of the most impressive epochs of human achievement,"[15] and he went on to outline what he considered to be the "twelve definitive moments" that form the major events of this period, beginning with the development of penicillin and other antibiotic compounds. As a result of these and other interventions, the western world has seen most infection removed from among the major causes of death, the total eradication of the one-time killer disease—smallpox—and the near eradication of poliomyelitis. It has seen major advances in the general prevention, diagnosis, and treatment of many of humanity's old enemies, especially in the development of surgical and other life-saving techniques from open heart surgery to organ transplants. Side by side with these developments, and some would argue, more importantly, have been major improvements in social conditions, particularly the provision of clean water supplies, adequate sewage systems, and improved diet, all of which together have produced, in the developed world, what is probably the longest lived, best fed, and safest society in human history. The vastly improved life expectancies of people in western society now mean that someone aged sixty-five years in 2011 may reasonably expect to live for more than another twenty years, and with a very good chance of becoming a centenarian.[16]

It might have been expected that the benefits of modern medicine would have brought about a reduction in the concerns of people over their general health and well-being. In fact, in spite of these improvements affecting all elements of western societies, the past few years have seen the growth of what may be termed an almost neurotic concern with issues of health and safety. Western society has become full of the "worried well" to the extent that normal, fit people are more worried about their health than they ever have been, a phenomenon partially fueled by a growing medical obsession with what, in real terms, are no more than imaginary dangers, dreamed up in often dubious epidemiological studies.[17]

15. Le Fanu, *Rise and Fall*, 1.
16. Department for Work and Pensions (UK), *Number*.
17. Skrabanek, *Death*.

Two parallel developments would appear to have accompanied this growth in people's concerns about their health. On the one hand, there has been a marked increase in public expectation of what conventional medicine is able to achieve, often fueled by exaggerated press reporting of new developments and discoveries. The successes of modern medical science have brought about false hopes and oftentimes unrealistic demands on the health services. The failure to meet these demands and expectations has frequently produced disappointment and disillusionment, which, in turn, has led people to turn to the alternative practitioners for help. In parallel with this, there has also been a growth in anti-scientific bias and an increasing "anti-doctor" stance that has been associated with the rise of nonconventional medical practice. This would seem to be part of that wider anti-scientific attitude that is a feature of what has been called "post-modern" thinking, a bias that was well illustrated by a comment of a theological writer, to the effect that the scientific and rational era of the twentieth century "has seeped over into the early twenty-first century."[18] One would have hoped that rational systems of thought would have been the norm, rather than something that had seeped over from a previous age. Nonetheless, rational thought has served the world well, and its detractors would do well to consider what life would be like today without the benefits it has provided over the past years. Once mystical conjecture has been allowed to infiltrate the way we think, then rational thought is in danger of being abandoned in favor of superstition and magic.

It is perhaps worth diverting slightly from the main issues in order to make some comment about the phenomenon of post-modern thought in view of the influence it has had on religious thinking in recent years. The term "post-modernism" was coined by the French philosopher Jean-Francois Lyotard, who considered its defining characteristic as incredulity towards meta-narratives, although this reflects but one aspect of a thought system that, in reality, is notoriously difficult to define. Someone remarked that as a system of thought it bears all the amorphous properties of jelly. Post-modernism is a general and wide-ranging term, applied to literature, art, philosophy, architecture, fiction, cultural and literary criticism, as well as to aspects of religious thought. Its roots lie, to a large extent, in the philosophies of Kierkegaard, Nietzsche, and Heidegger among others, and, in many ways, it may be seen as a reflection of the intense individualism that

---

18. Wainwright, *Spirit Possession*, 156.

is so much the dominant feature of western society. It is also a reflection of the underlying uncertainties of the modern world.

Most observers would agree that post-modernism may be understood as a reaction to the assumed certainty of scientific or other objective efforts to explain reality, and arises from an assumption that reality is not simply mirrored in the human understanding of it, but rather, is constructed as the individual attempts to understand his or her own particular and personal reality. For this reason, post-modernism rejects all meta-narratives and all explanations that claim universal validity. Instead, its focus is on the relative truths of each person. In the post-modern understanding, interpretation is everything. Reality only comes into being through our interpretations of what the world means to us individually; it is experience (fallible and relative though it may be) that provides the key to unlocking the door to one's personal truth. Scientific, philosophical, or religious truth is thus unable to provide universally valid explanations of reality. The paradox of the post-modern position is that, in placing all principles under the scrutiny of its skepticism, it must realize that even its own principles are not beyond questioning, for to argue that it is impossible to distinguish between true and false interpretations is to contradict oneself. Post-modernism is, in fact, entrapped by its own circular reasoning.

Post-modern philosophies, nonetheless, remain highly influential in spite of their inner contradictions, and it is likely that one of the reasons for this lies in the fact that they are not prepared to accept the overarching and all-explanatory narratives of either science or official religion. Science, it is argued, has led humanity into a cul-de-sac, and official, organized religion has led people into oppressive belief systems that have destroyed individual expression as well as personal expressions of "spirituality." Indeed, in the church itself, there has been a marked shift in thinking away from explicit Christian inspiration to notions of a vague "spirituality," that seems little more than the lowest common denominator of all religions or none. As noted above, the post-modern world discards the scientific worldview on the grounds that there can be no single explanation of all things, and instead "truth" becomes an internal frame of reference. Thus, it takes a pluralistic stance in which there is no final or absolute truth; the only guiding principle becomes "what is good for me." In this consumer-driven religious climate, a person's "spirituality" merely reflects the á la carte beliefs of the religious shopper. The warm fuzziness of much of alternative medical practice, consequently, has great appeal to those who follow this new philosophy of the consumer society.

At the same time, it has also to be said that it is very possible that some of the shift towards unorthodox medical practice has arisen from the hubris of the modern medical profession, and its tendency to be over-detached, and objective in the treatment of patients, as well as facing bureaucratic and institutional pressures to provide measurable outcomes for the benefit of the balance sheets. Further, the inevitable fragmentation of medical services, largely as a result of increasing specialization and ever diminishing financial resources, has tended to isolate the patient even more.

The alternative practitioner is not usually in this situation and tends to be able to devote more time and attention to the patient, appearing as more sympathetic to the underlying needs and problems. They tend to be great exponents of warmth, touch, and feeling, and a general comforting fuzziness in word and thought. As a result of the psychosocial dynamics of these practitioner/patient interactions, the patient feels better, even though the beneficial results of the different therapies are generally no different from placebo and need to be carefully differentiated from genuine "cure." It has to be said, however, that there is some evidence, although admittedly not well substantiated, that "feel-good" therapies may exert a generalized beneficial effect, also seen as a result of other situations in which there is an improvement in feelings of well-being. The old adage that "laughter is the best medicine" has an element of truth. When the patient feels better, there is a possibility that the response to proper medical treatment will be enhanced, in some cases at least, as a result of improved immune responses.[19] Feeling better, however, is a far cry from being cured of a disease, and alternative therapies do nothing for genuine pathology, other than, all too often, making it worse.

There is thus a wide diversity of differing approaches to the treatment of human illness. Modern scientific medicine is based on an increasing level of understanding of anatomy, physiology, and pathological processes, as well as biochemistry, pharmacology, and related disciplines, even though many of its advances have been the result of serendipity. Scientific medicine leads to the definition of the causes of disease in exact terms, identifying causal organisms, environmental factors, and so forth, even to the extent of being able to isolate specific genes as being the cause of certain conditions. The understandings of disease etiology have allowed for the development of equivalently exact forms of treatment, whether this be something as much taken for granted today as the prescription of the correct antibiotic

---

19. Keilcolt-Glaser, et al., "Psychoneuroimmunology," 15–28.

for an infection or the use of replacement hormones in various deficiency diseases such as diabetes.

At the other end of the spectrum from scientific medicine lie those various approaches to "healing" that run the whole gamut from folk medicine to magic. It is certainly true that some forms of empirical treatment can be shown to work, as in the case of certain herbal remedies, although they are not without their dangers, and they are often prescribed, not on any rational basis, but simply on an observation that they may work in certain circumstances. More dangerous, however, are the practitioners of what can only be called magico-religious medicine in which incantations, charms, and other "mumbo-jumbo" take the place of empirical or rational therapies.

It was observed, some years ago, that the "market for non-orthodox health care seems to be buoyant."[20] There is no sign that the situation is changing, and the hopes expressed by the British Medical Association that this "flight from science" was a "passing fashion"[21] show little sign of being realized. Alternative medicine, so-called, is alive and well and growing. As an aside, the "flight from science" seems to be true across the board, and not simply in medicine. What seems to be happening is the joining of various forms of new superstitions with remnants of the old, with the result that there is a growing trend for the world to become re-mystified rather than de-mystified, and that, in itself, is very much a feature of post-modern thinking. It seems very likely, therefore, that the growth of healing ministries in the church today, especially in respect of the more extreme forms of faith healing, is to be seen against this background of distrust of, and the general rise of alternatives to, scientific medicine and is not an isolated phenomenon in itself but a reflection of trends in modern western society.

The ancient Roman world, in which the young Christian congregations began and grew, was also characterized by very diverse approaches to the cure of disease. Credulity was widespread, and popular superstition and magical ideas persisted side by side with the more rational and scientific approach characterized by Greek and Roman medicine and associated with the names of Hippocrates, Galen, and others. It is a picture that does not seem so very different from today's western world in which rational concepts of disease, diagnosis, and treatment co-exist with quite irrational, and, at times, magical concepts. The attribution of disease to the work of demons, as found in some religious groups, together with the use of magic

20. Thomas, et al., "Use of Non-orthodox," 207–10.
21. Board of Science, *Alternative Therapies*.

and superstition among so-called "New Age" practitioners, are examples of the widespread credulity that can exist in a scientific age. It is always possible to hold mutually exclusive ideas together with apparent ease, rather like Lewis Carroll's White Queen (in *Through the Looking Glass*) who boasted of being able to believe six impossible things before breakfast.[22] The fact is, however, that both sets of postulates cannot be right—a disease may not be caused by both a bacterium or an internal chemical imbalance on the one hand, and an evil spirit or other spiritual cause on the other. One or other of the causal postulates has to be wrong. The all-too-frequent human tragedies occur when credulous people believe the spiritual causation to be correct and ignore or refuse proper medical care. Ministers of the church have not been without blame in fostering such behavior. I refer to this aspect of so-called "healing ministry" as the "unacceptable face of healing," and it will be discussed in detail later in chapter 5.

The growth of alternative medical practice, often of a very dubious nature, raises the interesting question of why it is that there should be this search for non-scientific models of healing, frequently based on irrational, and, at times, nonsensical, concepts of reality. Why are some people attracted to the irrational, whereas the majority of people are generally satisfied with the medical model of the cure of a disease process based on rational concepts of pathology and therapy? It is a question outside the limits of this study, but it does raise the further question of what is really meant by the word "healing."

HEALING—A SLIPPERY WORD

At the outset of this study, the inherent difficulty of defining the term "healing" in an adequate manner was noted. The word is used so loosely in a variety of contexts that one is frequently reminded of Lewis Carroll's Humpty Dumpty, who remarked to Alice (in *Alice's Adventures in Wonderland*) in a somewhat scornful tone, "When *I* use a word it means just what I choose it to mean—neither more nor less."[23] Healing is not a word often used in orthodox medical practice except with certain quite specific meanings, such as the healing of wounds or ulcers, for example. As John Wilkinson once noted, "we shall find chapters on healing in books about alternative medicine and references to healing in articles by doctors whose medical

22. Carroll, *Through the Looking Glass*, 207.
23. Carroll, *Alice in Wonderland*, 222.

orthodoxy is often in doubt. So much so, that for many doctors healing is synonymous with quackery. In other words, healing is to be distinguished from the orthodox practice of medicine and the word is not used in polite circles."[24] Medical practitioners who deal with discrete pathological processes would generally tend to use words such as "cure" or "remission."

The inherent ambiguity of the word "healing" is compounded by the very different understandings that exist, both of the nature of health and healing, as well as the methods by which healing may be brought about. The whole forms a good example of Wittgenstein's well-known dictum that "the meaning is the use"; and, in the world of spiritual healing, both meaning and use may be stretched far beyond any rational understanding of the word. The problem is that unless one has been initiated into the underlying philosophy and presuppositions behind the "use," it becomes extremely difficult to grasp the actual "meaning" that is being conveyed. The Healing Trust in the United Kingdom, an umbrella organization for a large number of "spiritual healers," defines healing as the regaining of the balance of mind, body, and/or emotions. Such a definition is so broad as to become virtually meaningless, and reminds one of the ancient belief in the balance of the humors as the basis of good health.

The whole matter is further compounded in those vague and woolly areas of healing practice covered by such terms as the "healing of memories," and other forms of what is referred to as "inner healing." In these categories the use of the word healing becomes essentially metaphorical, and relates solely to the induction of some form of religious feeling of well-being. It certainly has nothing to do with the healing of physical disease, although in loose terms such practices may represent a form of psychotherapy, and consequently may be of some benefit to the recipient, particularly in psychosomatic illness. At the very least, however, such usage is indeterminate. The usual, in fact, what one might call the common sense, understanding of what would generally be understood as "healing," is perhaps even more misrepresented when centers for the care of the terminally ill are called "healing centers." Healing, in any normal use of the word, is somewhat unlikely, to say the least, for someone dying of a terminal illness. The practice is defended, nonetheless, on the specious, and quite extraordinary argument, that "healing" may occur through death! One is reminded of the words of Sir Walter Raleigh about the headman's axe that was soon

---

24. Wilkinson, "Healing," 17–37.

to end his life, that it was a sure cure for all diseases! However, one cannot but consider that Humpty Dumpty certainly seems to be having a field day!

These vaguer areas of so-called healing practice, although they are increasingly to be found in religious circles, will not be further discussed, as by their very nature they defy proper categorization and quantification. Studies have shown that so-called healing rituals may often provide immediate, but usually transient, beneficial effects in improving feelings of well-being,[25] but that is very different from the claims for the physical cure of specific illness, the examination of which is the main thrust of this study. Consequently, it is the basic assumption in all that follows, that the term "healing," when used in a medical context and relating to sick people must include the reality of the physical cure of disease, measurable by the use of the proper criteria, otherwise the term becomes meaningless, and reasonable discussion impossible.

In the chapters that follow I will attempt to examine the modern healing movement in general terms, with particular emphasis on faith healing as practiced notably by the followers of charismatic renewal. I will also give some consideration to other forms of healing practice, including the claims arising from shrines such as Lourdes, from those who practice so-called "sacramental healing," as well as considering the effectiveness of intercessory prayer on the course of physical pathology. The primary aim of the study, therefore, is to examine what evidence exists for the effectiveness of religious healing practices in an attempt to answer the vital question of whether any form of spiritual healing actually results in the genuine cure of physical disease; in other words, does it work? In addition, I will also give some attention to the numerous disasters that have followed in the wake of healing ministry, what I have called, "the unacceptable face of healing," particularly, although not exclusively, as a result of exorcisms, and so-called deliverance ministry. Rather than leave such a study without suggesting a way forward out of the conflicting claims and counter-claims, the final chapter will give some thought to an alternative approach for the church's ministry to the sick and needy, that emphasizes the much more demanding requirement of pastoral care within the overall task of what used to be called, very appropriately, "the cure of souls."

---

25. Ness and Wintrobe, "Emotional Impact," 302–15; and Glik, "Psychosocial," 579–86.

2

Basic Approaches
Complementary or Alternative?

THE SUPERMARKET SHOPPING TROLLEY represents, perhaps, the abiding symbol of every aspect of the modern consumer society. Personal choice is all important, and it is not altogether surprising that there exists a wide range of alternatives to the standard practice of scientific medicine. The boxes into which these various options are usually placed are generally labelled "complementary" or "alternative," terms that have already been used in this study. It is rather unfortunate that these two terms are often used interchangeably, as there seems little doubt that a distinction should be drawn between them in terms of the relationship of their practitioners to orthodox medical treatment. There is, after all, a very real difference between someone who wishes to provide a form of therapy that is designed to replace the treatment offered by a registered medical practitioner, and a person who wishes merely to offer something additional, as support or an ancillary therapy, designed to complement what the doctor provides. The problem has arisen, however, that many of those associated with the Christian healing movement have tended to cross the boundaries and become involved with attempts to "cure" disease rather than simply offering care and support for the sufferer. In other words, what should have remained "complementary" has instead become an "alternative." In this chapter, therefore, consideration will be given to those whose ministrations tend to form an alternative to medical practice, as well as to those who wish simply to complement normal treatment measures with a ministry that is designed to meet the wider psycho-social and spiritual needs of the patient, especially those with serious or terminal illness.

COMPLEMENTARY MINISTRIES

Those who are involved in forms of religious healing that may be considered as complementary to normal medical treatment, with the use of intercessory prayer, the laying on of hands, anointing, and other support mechanisms for the patient, will very often consider that their ministry constitutes a form of "spiritual healing." At the same time, however, it would generally be true to say that they would not wish their ministrations to be seen as being in opposition to normal medical practice, nor would they wish to undermine a patient's faith in standard medical therapy. It would be normal for them to encourage patients to seek medical help for their illnesses, but, in addition, they would also consider that their work offered a dimension of the total curative process that would be missing from the disease-specific treatment provided by a medical practitioner, although possibly being no more than a significant level of social, psychological, and spiritual support. Those healers falling within this group would be, for example, those who subscribe to the strict codes of ethics and conduct of such bodies as the British Confederation of Healing Organizations, which represents over 7,000 "healers" with a wide range of beliefs, not all Christian by any means, as well as those involved in such organizations as the Order of St Luke the Physician, an ecumenical society that recognizes the importance of normal medical and surgical treatment, and promotes co-operation with the medical profession, while at the same time, emphasizing the importance of the spiritual dimension.

Organizations of this type are very concerned to exclude charlatans, and make it clear that the "healing" they offer is not medical aid as defined by law, but rather is simply the beneficial effect that the healer's administrations may have on the patient, particularly in respect of the psyche. These practitioners thus make a distinction between what is to be seen as "cure" as a result of normal therapeutic measures, and what they call "healing," something that belongs to a wider dimension, and produces effects on the general well-being and the restoration of the whole person rather than simply on a specific, and possibly limited, pathological process.

Basic Approaches

It is likely that the majority of those involved in the church's healing ministry would be characterized by this approach, and their primary aim would be to offer prayer and pastoral support to those who are sick without making any substantive claims about the possible curative effectiveness of their prayers. Such forms of ministry undoubtedly have short-term beneficial effects, mainly in the form of enhanced feelings of well-being. The long term and permanent benefits of such ministrations, however, remain unproven. Nonetheless, the fact that these practitioners do not seek to provide an alternative therapy to standard medical practice means that their work is to be regarded as an acceptable adjunct to normal medical treatment, and, at least as far as the patient is concerned, it may well provide valuable psycho-social, and indeed, in the context of Christian (or other religious) pastoral ministry, spiritual benefits for the patient.

Essentially, the benefits of these forms of ministry may be understood as what is called the "placebo effect,"[1] that is the beneficial effect on a person's symptoms as a result of the administration of something that has no real effect on the underlying disease process, but which, through mental processes, has the ability to relieve symptoms, although without affecting any underlying pathology. It has been shown that even though placebos do not act on the disease, they do have an effect on the relief of symptoms in about one in three patients. In most cases, however, the effect lasts for a short time only, and is probably a result of the body's own ability to relieve pain and other symptoms as a result of the stimulation of the body's immune system, and the release of various chemical compounds through the brain's activity. It is likely that there is more than a single mechanism involved, and there are possibly multiple effects with differing neurobiological pathways.[2] However, even though the exact mechanism of the placebo effect may not be known, the awareness that the mind can affect the body has been part of folk medicine for many years. These links were well known in ancient cultures as well as in various methods of folk medicine today, and many forms of treatment provided by shamans or medicine men depended on these mind–body connections, and were often effective because of the patient's strong belief in the healing power and methods of the shaman. The shaman himself, however, would not have viewed his efforts as placebos, but as effective methods of treatment.

---

1. Shapiro and Shapiro, *The Powerful Placebo*; Kaptchuk, "The Placebo Effect," 817–25, and Wampold, et al., "The Placebo is Powerful," 835–54.

2. Finniss et al., "Placebo Effects," 686–95.

On the other hand, it is possible that the sick person was going to get better, irrespective of any form of treatment, as a consequence of the natural history of the condition and the ability of the body to heal itself. The recovery was thought to be because of the treatment, although, in fact, it had done very little towards the cure of the illness.

The use of placebos is not restricted to folk medicine, on the one hand, nor alternative therapies, on the other. It is likely that most doctors at some time in their practice have used placebos to relieve certain symptoms such as pain, anxiety, and trouble sleeping in some of their patients.[3] There are occasions when placebos have been given by doctors out of feelings of frustration or even desperation, because nothing else seemed likely to work. In a study published in 2008, for example, nearly half of physicians who responded to the poll said that they used a placebo when they felt that it might help the patient feel better.[4] Those words are important. As a result of using a placebo, the patient felt better, and it will be noted later in this study that this is a not uncommon response to the effects of the application of religious healing rites. If the patient believes in the treatment and wants it to work, it can seem to do so, at least for a while. This is not the same, however, as being cured in the sense of a curative effect on the underlying pathology of the disease.

The distinction that many of those involved in religious healing make between "cure" and "healing" derives from their conviction that the former is essentially incomplete in itself, and that the whole person needs to return to "health," in whatever way that may be defined. Many orthodox medical practitioners would have few problems with such an understanding in broad terms, and the traditional role of the church in caring for the sick in both physical and spiritual support may be seen as a form of complementary therapy, involving co-operation between clergy and/or lay church people on the one hand, and the medical profession on the other, providing a ministry to the whole person. Provided that the church's ministry was restricted to such an integrative approach, with an emphasis on care and support, there could be few arguments against it, although it would be better termed a "caring" ministry rather than a "healing" ministry, belonging properly to the "cure of souls," rather than the cure of bodies. Unfortunately, most so-called "healing ministries" have adopted a much wider approach than a pastoral ministry, and, all too often, they would see themselves in the

3. Brody and Miller, "Lessons," 2612–13.
4. Sherman and Hickner, "Academic Physicians," 7–10.

business of "curing," rather than simply assisting in the "healing" process, in the sense that this term has been used in the foregoing discussion.

Furthermore, even in those situations where the proper boundaries of the church's role have been observed, there has been very little in the way of genuine co-operation between clergy, and the medical profession, with both clergy and lay ministers acting independently of doctors and other health professionals, and often with no real knowledge of the patient's condition, and more particularly, with no proper understanding of the diagnosis. It is worth adding that patients themselves often have no proper understanding of the diagnosis or nature of their condition, and consequently, the information they pass to their ministers or priests will frequently be inadequate, and often wrong, which does not make for an effective intervention by the religious healer.

SACRAMENTAL HEALING PRACTICES

It would be a general experience that, in all religions, prayer for the sick tends to be prayer for the cure of the patient, rather than simply supportive pastoral prayer for those specific matters that are more strictly the concern of the religious community, such as spiritual welfare and general psychosocial support. In Christian circles this judgment would be true across the board, not only in respect of those forms of healing ministries that openly claim to provide cures, such as those associated with the pentecostal and charismatic movements, but also among churches generally and, more particularly perhaps, among those who practice what may be termed "sacramental healing." It needs to be said, however, that sacramental healing practices are generally far removed from the charismatic style of religious healing and would be broadly classified as complementary rather than alternative. It is a religious approach to sickness that has a long history and is to be found primarily in those church communities having a strong liturgical tradition, such as Roman Catholic, Anglican, and Lutheran circles, as well as the Eastern Orthodox churches.

Sacramental healing is an approach to ministry to the sick that has seen a major resurgence in popularity, particularly in the Anglican communion since the 1920s, and its development has been detailed by Mews[5] and Gusmer.[6] This growth of interest in religious healing has led to significant

5. Mews, "Revival," 229–331.
6. Gusmer, *Ministry of Healing*.

changes in liturgy, to the development of religious healing centers, and to attempts at interdisciplinary dialogue with the medical profession. Initially there was an emphasis on healing practices being in the hands of ordained ministers with the necessary training, although this has changed considerably so that lay members of congregations will now often be closely involved. There is an undoubted problem with this as it is by no means certain that laypeople have adequate awareness of the need for complete confidentiality in their dealings with sick people.

A number of strong moves that took place at that time saw the introduction of anointing and the imposition of hands into the 1928 revision of the Church of England's *Book of Common Prayer*. In fact, this revision was never authorized, but it was frequently used, and its revisions of previous liturgical practice became widely accepted so that a "Form of Unction and the Laying on of Hands" was approved for provisional use in 1935. These revisions were introduced because the existing service for the visitation of the sick was considered to be both theologically and pastorally inadequate, and they became the jumping-off point for the more radical changes that were to take place in later years.

The New Zealand Anglican Prayer Book of 1988, revised in 1997 and again in 2002 (*A New Zealand Prayer Book/He Karakia Mihinare o Aotearoa*) is a good example of the changes that have come about, almost imperceptibly, from traditional practice. In its pastoral liturgies, it has a specific section devoted to "The Ministry of Healing," associated with sacramental anointing. Similar liturgies have appeared elsewhere in recent years, for example in the revised *Book of Common Prayer* of the American Episcopal Church (1979), and the *Book of Common Worship* of the Church of England (2001). It is of note that liturgies of anointing or unction had no place in the earlier formularies such as the 1662 *Book of Common Prayer*, which is effectively the basis of all later arising Anglican prayer books. The use of anointing (unction), in fact, was specifically abolished in Reformation times and was not to be found in any of the authorized prayer books, apart from a short-lived liturgy for the anointing of the sick in Cranmer's first Prayer Book of 1549. It vanished in the 1551 revision, never to reappear until the twentieth century, under the influence of what was essentially Anglo-Catholic thinking, and largely borrowed from Roman Catholic practice.

The wording of these new liturgies, all of which make provision both for the laying on of hands and for anointing, is such that it would appear to suggest that this ministry of healing takes the form of an "alternative" to medical practice, with an apparent underlying claim that the actual anointing is expected to do something for the sick person rather than provide comfort and support. Indeed, these liturgies have been described as "therapeutic rites," a terminology that would seem to indicate that the processes of prayer and anointing are somehow expected to convey some tangible and real value, beyond what might be expected in terms of their spiritual value to the sick person. An examination of the wording of these liturgies makes it clear that the actions are to convey healing, and there would seem to be little doubt that they are meant to be more than symbolic. They clearly express an understanding that something is being conveyed to the sick, the purpose of which is to bring them back to health.

The anointing of the sick in the Roman Catholic Church has been considered as a sacrament of the church at least from the time of Peter Lombard in the twelfth century. It continues the older practice of extreme unction, in that it is largely reserved for the very sick, and those nearing the end of life, unlike the common practice of other communions. It still carries with it, in essence, much of the thinking behind the old rite, although there have been considerable changes since Vatican II. The purpose is expressed in the *Catechism of the Catholic Church* (2nd ed., 1997) as "the conferral of a special grace on the Christian experiencing the difficulties of grave illness or old age." It is interesting, however, that there is far less emphasis on bodily healing than in the Anglican rites. The Roman Catholic Church believes that the Dominical charge to heal the sick remains in operation, but the major emphasis of the rite is on the remission of sins, and its purpose is to lead the sick person to healing of the soul, and only of the body if such is God's will. Physical healing is not assumed in this rite, and the major function of the rite would be to confer sanctifying grace sacramentally.

It is suggested that in all liturgies of this general form there seems to be an underlying understanding that the act of anointing works by an inherent power that enables it to confer a grace that is somehow resident in the act itself. It comes perilously close to magic and the revival of an understanding of the sacraments as effective *ex opere operato*, that it to say, efficacious in and of themselves. It is almost as though grace was something to be poured out when the stopper was removed. Grace in biblical terms, however, is always relational. In the New Testament, grace is centered in Christ and is the expression of the unconditional love of God that Christ mediates to the world. It could be argued, in fact, that grace is possibly not even an appropriate word to use in respect of the value to the recipient of the historic

Christian sacraments of baptism and holy communion, although centuries of use would make it impossible to change the practice. Whatever spiritual value actions such as anointing may have for the individual, it is important to recognize that it is derived from the belief of the recipient in that value, not because of something done by the person administering the rite; in other words, any beneficial effect is a placebo effect. Should the dramatic actions of the Christian sacraments result in a greater appreciation of God's grace in Christ, then it becomes reasonable to speak of them as "means of grace," always with the recognition that any meaning they may have is dependent exclusively upon the belief of the participant in their effectiveness. Religious actions, such as the practice of anointing the sick, whether or not they are designated sacramental, are not magically operative rites and do not have any quality of efficacy in themselves or by themselves.

Although religious actions will be associated with beneficial effects for the sick believer in providing support and a sense of spiritual well-being, such moral and spiritual effects do not constitute "cure." Furthermore, the established rituals of anointing the sick tend to perpetuate the cruel myth of a causal link between sickness and sin, and this alone raises concerns about their propriety. Making a causal link between disease and a failure to meet religious and moral obligations has been a feature of probably most religions, and in some sense it may be seen as an attempt to answer the unanswerable question, "Why me?" Contagious and disfiguring diseases, of which the best example is the disease complex unfortunately called leprosy in most English translations of the Bible, were particularly liable to be understood as direct punishments for some form of transgression. Various ritual prescriptions were applied to these diseases in order to avoid the contamination of the community, which was seen as more important than the healing of the sick person. In consequence, consulting a physician for help could be construed as a denial of the primary role of God and evidence of lack of faith in him, as well as a lack of willingness to acknowledge personal sin (note 2 Chron 16:12).

It was these concepts that were carried over and perpetuated in Christianity, even though such a simplistic viewpoint had been challenged in the Bible (for example, in the book of Job in the Hebrew Bible and John 9:1–3 in the New Testament). The early church, however, persisted with such ideas, possibly through the vested interests of a growing clerical caste, and medical treatment was displaced by an emphasis on prayer and fasting in order to chasten the individual. From the Renaissance onward, however,

Basic Approaches

medical practice and the church became increasingly divorced from one another, allowing the development of medicine along the now familiar lines of scientific principles from the sixteenth or seventeenth centuries onward. Nonetheless, the church has always believed that it had a valid role in ministering to the sick. In general, this has not been considered to be in competition with orthodox medicine, but rather as complementary to it. Some of the more recent developments in healing ministries, however, particularly those associated with pentecostal churches and the charismatic movement, seem to be drifting towards a return to a pre-scientific worldview (one notes particularly the emphasis on demonic possession) and inevitably this will be in conflict with modern medical practice.

The biblical basis for anointing the sick is derived essentially from the New Testament letter of James. The directions set out in James 5:14–16 form a sort of prototype for the anointing of sick people, and consequently provided a ready-made basis for practice within Christian churches. It is suggested, however, that a more considered examination of this passage will set out a somewhat different understanding, and point rather to a theology of healing that is quite specifically directed towards a restoration of church members with non-physical conditions, that is to say with problems of mood and emotion.[7] The treatment of these conditions requires what may be called a psychological approach, and the directions for the prayers and administrations of the church elders given in the letter of James provided the right dynamics, particularly through confession of sins and assurance of forgiveness, to produce a therapeutic environment enabling the sufferer of certain very specific types of condition to make progress towards recovery.

There can be no reasonable doubt, however, that in this specific passage, anointing itself is not understood as being curative, but is simply a symbolic action illustrating the care and support, both of the congregation and also of God. Similarly, in the modern situation, whatever psychological value the act of anointing may have for the patient, it cannot be seen as either necessary or effectual by itself. Neither, for that matter, may the "prayer of faith" be understood as some special miracle-working prayer that can act like magic. God does not act in an arbitrary manner to rearrange the molecules of the human body. What he does do is to give meaning to the present reality of existence, and within that boundary, prayer, with or without

---

7. I have discussed this in detail in both my studies of New Testament healing; see Howard, *Disease and Healing*, 259–66; Howard, *Medicine, Miracle and Myth*, 97–99; and briefly in chapter 1. My conclusions owe much to Wright, "Healing," 20–21.

associated anointing, may have meaning for the individual as an assurance of God's love in difficult circumstances. In real terms, the effects are on the mind, and where there is strong belief, that belief can provide varying degrees of relief from whatever it is that ails the sufferer.

Nonetheless, whether intentionally or not, the modern rituals of healing and anointing seem to present an understanding of disease that owes more to medieval thought than it does to the concepts of the twenty-first century. Religious rites seem to be understood as having curative powers, and the formularies do not provide any suggestion that the function of religious ministry is simply to stand beside, and be supportive of, normal medical treatment. Equally, and I think very importantly, there is no indication that such normal medical treatment is likely to be the only effective means of bringing about the cure of the sick person suffering from organic disease. Further, and perhaps significantly, it is also to be noted that nowhere in these liturgies are there any prayers for wisdom and understanding for those who provide the therapeutic and caring services of medicine that, in the final analysis, are likely to be the sole providers of cure.

It is reasonable to suppose, however, that the majority of those who are involved with the practices of laying on of hands, and anointing the sick would be unlikely to discredit the place of normal medical practice in their ministry, at least one would sincerely hope so, particularly in view of the increasing numbers of laypeople, rather than properly trained members of the clergy, involved in these practices. On the other hand, there are those groups within the church (and also in non-Christian circles, let it be said) who do see their activities as being real alternatives to medical practice, and they will frequently attempt to exclude normal curative medicine from any place in the treatment of illness, and will intentionally attempt to dissuade others from having recourse to doctors. The practitioners of Christian Science have been historically the group most marked by these attitudes, but such attitudes are also prominent in many pentecostal and charismatic groups, and mainline churches that have been strongly influenced by the charismatic movement, and it is to these groupings that I will now turn my attention.

Basic Approaches

THE CHARISMATIC TRADITION AND OTHER ALTERNATIVE PRACTITIONERS

A high proportion of the practitioners of so-called alternative medicine, as opposed to its many users, may be categorized as "religious" in broad terms. Apart from those advocating herbs, nutritional supplements, and other over-the-counter remedies, there are those "healers" associated with Christian charismatic congregationsm, and others who are grounded in the extensive range of philosophies of what is generally called the "New Age" movement with its various forms of "spirituality." This latter group use a wide variety of adjunct techniques, such as healing crystals, color therapy, iridology, and other measures that can only be called "hocus pocus," although they may provide some degree of psychological benefit to those who believe in them. It would have to be said, however, that many of those who believe in the value of "alternatives" to normal medical practice have essentially been indoctrinated by the "fear mongers" intent on selling their wares, like the pedlars of cure-all nostrums at a medieval fair. The really dangerous among these people are those who claim to see themselves as specially gifted by God and able to perform miracles that can cure even terminal illness. What makes these people particularly dangerous is that very often they themselves actually believe in their methods. It is well known that the Christian Science movement forbids its members to have any contact with medical practice, but outside such very clearly non-orthodox Christian groupings, both pentecostal churches and the various charismatic groups, either in the mainstream denominations or in independent congregations, have a pattern of anti-medical bias and advocate "faith healing" of various forms in opposition to, or certainly as an alternative to, normal medical treatment.

The charismatic renewal movement, although sharing in many of the attitudes and general ideas of the earlier pentecostalism, erupted as a unique phenomenon in the 1960s. In terms of its emphasis on healing, the movement was characterized by a failure to give proper medical treatment its due place, a warped spiritual warfare theology that re-introduced concepts such as demon possession as the cause of disease, and a false triumphalism that tried to avoid the recognition of suffering as part of normal human experience. Leaders of these congregations frequently make no secret of their antipathy and opposition to the use of standard medical procedures on the part of their followers. They argue that this would be showing evidence of disobedience and unfaithfulness, as well as demonstrating a sinful lack of faith. Some of the disastrous results of these attitudes are discussed in chapter 5.

Many of the emphases of these charismatic groups seem to be little different from those of the New Age movement with activities that seem to be far from the teachings of the New Testament and traditional orthodox Christianity. What is clear, however, is that all these forms of "healing" have had a long and colorful history, and the methods used are by no means specifically Christian. Indeed, much of what passes as spiritual healing in a Christian context is no different from other forms of religious healing systems throughout the world and may be regarded as a form of shamanism, discussed in detail by Lewis.[8] That patients may sometimes benefit from such practices is not in doubt, especially those with minor psychiatric conditions or suffering from non-specific chronic pain and similar disorders where there is a major psychological component. Once again, however, the effects are generally temporary and are essentially the result of the placebo effect. There is no removal of underlying physical pathology where this co-exists with the psychological problems.

Some care needs to be exercised in making broad judgments about charismatic and similar practices since the charismatic movement, in particular, is not easy to characterize in exact terms, and it is remarkably diverse in its various expressions, showing a wide spectrum of both thought and practice. Nonetheless, while many charismatic Christians would be happy to use the provisions of orthodox, scientific medicine, in addition to any spiritual ministry they may obtain from their churches, it is also clear that there is a substantial number who would look to what is termed "faith" as the sole medium of healing, and would, in fact, adopt an attitude little different from the practitioners of Christian Science, totally eschewing all forms of modern medicine. Adherents of these views appear to demonstrate a form of what someone called "cultural schizophrenia," attempting to hold to the naiveté of the biblical worldview on the one hand, while, at the same time, living normally in a scientific age and enjoying most of the benefits that science and technology have brought. Unfortunately, the basic presuppositions about the world held by older societies do not mix with a scientific worldview, and the attempt to live in both worlds produces incoherence and confusion.

The variety and complexity of the various alternatives offered by the charismatic movement almost defy description, and any attempt to provide

8. Lewis, *Ecstatic Religion*.

a detailed survey is impossible in a short study. Further, trying to delineate such diverse practices is to enter an entirely different world from that of rational modern medicine and scientific thought, an issue that Hexham has discussed in some detail.[9] The range of alternatives is bewildering, but this widespread return to practices often bordering on magic, is paralleled by the growth of other non-rational attitudes in society, to be seen, for example, in those associated with the more extreme elements of the environmental movement. The widespread fear of synthetic chemicals in western society is a good example of this phenomenon. It shows itself in what may be called "chemophobia," a fixed attitude of mind that totally ignores the fact that many naturally occurring chemicals are far more potent in their effects than anything normally produced or used in industry. Naturally occurring compounds, especially those from plant and fungal sources, which are much more abundant and widespread in the environment than industrial chemicals, are frequently more potent carcinogens or have much greater general toxicity than their industrial counterparts.

These attitudes of mind owe much to what has been termed "para-science," the development of a chain of circumstantial reasoning, often based on the manipulation and distortion of scientific half-truths, producing hypotheses that are generally not amenable to formal testing procedures, and which become, to all intents and purposes, something akin to oracles and thus, articles of faith. Reason has been abandoned. The process is reminiscent of the Bellman in Lewis Carroll's, *The Hunting of the Snark*, who told his crew, "I have said it thrice, what I tell you three times is true."[10] The "Bellman fallacy" is widespread in modern society, leading to these unsupported hypotheses rapidly gaining the status of fact. Then, in spite of all contrary evidence, they become established as articles of faith to their adherents, and to a large proportion of the general population as well, that lacks the knowledge to be able to make the necessary informed judgments. I have discussed these issues in detail elsewhere.[11]

It seems likely that there are two major factors that have fueled the growing interest in alternative approaches to the treatment of illness. Firstly, there is the increasing lack of any underlying certainties in modern western society. The modern world seems to lack the comfort of a well-ordered universe running on the tramlines of its predetermined course. Newtonian

---

9. Hexham, "Some Aspects," 415–29.
10. Carroll, *Hunting*. Fit the First, Stanza 2.
11. Howard, "Metals and Man," 403–10; and Howard, "Chemical Residues," 27–33.

physics gave way to quantum physics, and people have come to believe in a natural world that seems to be governed by chance and uncertainty rather than rigid natural laws. In point of fact, however, as Stephen Hawking put it, "[S]cience seems to have uncovered a set of laws that, within the limits set by the uncertainty principle, tell us how the universe will develop with time."[12] In other words, the universe continues to follow an ordered, rather than an arbitrary, path through time, and the rules still exist but are differently configured from the way in which they were conceived earlier, before Einstein, and those who have followed him.

Nonetheless, people have undoubtedly had difficulty in coming to terms with the revolutions in scientific thought, and the uncertainty surrounding our place in the universe, together with the effects of two world wars and political upheaval; and these factors have led to an undermining of the moral, philosophical, and religious certainties of previous generations. The result has been a climate of uncertainty and a crisis of confidence in science as the provider of answers to the day-to-day problems of human society, and in religion (at least in its organized forms) as the arbiter of moral decision-making. It has been inevitable that scientific medicine has suffered from this same crisis of confidence. Although people clamor for the great benefits of modern medicine in terms of the technological advances, particularly in surgical techniques, there is at the same time a distrust of the advances that have been made in other areas, especially in the applications of genetic science, reproductive technologies, and the use of the highly powerful therapeutic agents now available. Patients are often afraid of modern medicines, and the purveyors of the alternative therapies strike a responsive chord in the minds of many people. The apparent certainty of the fundamentalist, whether religious or secular, provides a much sought after security, even though it is generally false and fallible.

A second factor that has fed the growth of alternative medical practice has been the widening gap between the medical and lay perspectives on sickness and health. There is a very real difference between the scientific biomedical model of disease, based on discrete pathological processes, whether they be the activity of micro-organisms, age-related degeneration, or the uncontrolled growth of tumor cells, and the awareness and understanding of patients about their illness or sickness, that is, the way in which the disease process is experienced and understood by them. Scientific understandings may be (or at least often appear to

12. Hawking, *A Brief History*, 129.

be) reductionist, and they are in marked contrast to the understanding of the individual's "illness," as that is experienced in subjective terms of pain, weakness, and other forms of distress. Even should the patient have a scientific education, the subjective experience of illness will usually be given meaning outside the strict biomedical model of disease and pathology. Doctors often forget this, and are seen as distanced from the patient and lacking in empathy and understanding. It is greatly to be lamented that the modern emphasis on the science of medicine has lessened the practice of the art of medicine for far too many modern doctors, to the detriment of their patients' well-being. The well-known summary of the vocation of the doctor, attributed (probably wrongly) to the nineteenth-century pioneer in the treatment of tuberculosis, E. L. Trudeau, "*guérir quelquefois, soulager souvent, consoler toujours*" ("cure sometimes, relieve often, comfort always") has all too often been forgotten, ignoring the need to comfort in the rush to cure. It has been remarked that "physiological measurement, although an essential aspect of medicine, only gives one view about the complexity of human illness. The importance of patients' health beliefs should not be underestimated, especially since non-medical health care from family and friends still copes with most symptoms in the community."[13] These differences also tend to heighten the distinction between the ideas of cure and healing in the popular mind.

Many factors are thus likely to be at work in helping to determine, or at least influence, the ways in which people deal with their illnesses, as well as the sort of people to whom they turn for help. What is important to remember throughout this discussion, however, is the fact that, for all its failures, it is scientific medicine alone that is genuinely open to an experimental testing of its claims. It is, in fact, this openness to falsification that is the mark of genuine science, and it is this approach that is the basis of modern "evidence-based" medicine. What makes scientific theories worthy of serious attention is not that there are good grounds for believing their truth, but that they are open to experimental refutation. The problem with the various claims made by the practitioners of alternative medicine in its many forms—and in the specific context of this study, those of the healing movement in the church—is that, in general, they are not open to testing methods, and their practitioners would largely reject the appropriateness of such testing for evaluating their claims. This has been particularly the case in a religious context where the need for adequate evidence for the claims of

13. Helman, "Limits," 1080–83.

success in healing has been viewed as almost blasphemous. As Larry Briskman once put it, "what renders the theories of witchcraft, scientology, and so on unworthy of serious consideration from the point of view of truth is not that there do not exist 'good empirical grounds' for believing their truth (such 'grounds' exist for every theory), but rather that they are immune to any attempt to refute them empirically, or if they are not so immune, are easily refuted as soon as the attempt is made."[14] It is interesting, however, that even when an alternative therapy is shown to be valueless, there is little if any change in behavior in those who have used it. Since the 1990s, the United States National Institutes for Health have spent (some would argue, wasted) millions of dollars in testing various forms of alternative medicine; but in spite of demonstrating their lack of effectiveness in the treatment of disease, there is remarkable little evidence for any changes in behavior in the American public.[15]

The foregoing considerations, although they have done no more than touch the surface of the complex issues involved, provide the basis for the remaining chapters in which I will look at the main approaches to Christian healing practice, and the evidence for its effectiveness. In the process there will also be a passing look at what I have called "the unacceptable face of healing," the stories of some of the sad cases of people, including children and the mentally ill, who, as a result of misguided faith in so-called "healers," whose practices promised much, but delivered little, were made far worse rather than better.

14. Briskman, "Doctors and Witchdoctors," 1108–10.
15. Offit, "Studying Complementary," 1803–4.

3

Healing In Practice

THE IMPORTANCE OF "FAITH," a term not always sufficiently defined, as the essential prerequisite for effective healing has been central to the practice of all forms of religious healing, from the past to the present. This was true of the ministry of Jesus, which was reported on at least one occasion to have failed through the lack of faith of the townspeople (Mark 6:1–6). It was equally true among the very different branches of the Christian church that developed healing practices at various times in their history, and, more specifically, it remains true in relation to such ministries in churches today. In addition to this emphasis, there is generally a remnant of those earlier negative attitudes towards sickness that understood it as being in some way the result of sin, attitudes that developed from the late classical period onwards, in which medical treatment was displaced, in Christian religious thought, by an emphasis on prayer and fasting to chasten the individual. Even in the service for the Visitation of the Sick in the 1662 *Book of Common Prayer* of the Church of England there is a strong emphasis on the need for the sick person to repent and receive absolution. The service states explicitly that sickness is "God's visitation," either because of sin or to provide testing and trial of the individual. It provides, in fact, a good illustration of the point that I have made elsewhere that, "until there was any proper understanding of the causative factors in disease and the actual disease processes themselves, there was a tendency to see sickness as the result of divine visitations and punishment for wrongdoing."[1]

Although rational theories of disease causation existed in earlier times, such as the understanding that disease came from disturbances in the balance of the "humors," the church consistently tended to foster an attitude that linked disease with a failure to meet one's religious and moral obligations, an approach that has been fostered in perhaps most religions over human history. One might observe that to foster these links and lay emphasis on human failure and sin will continue to provide clergy or other religious leaders with a central and unassailable position, as it is only they who have the authority to forgive sins on God's behalf, and therefore bring relief to the sufferer. An element of vested interest, therefore, may be partly responsible for the continuance of these ideas.

It is certainly unfortunate that these concepts persist into the present time, and virtually all the writings of Christian authors on the subject of spiritual/faith healing emphasize that individual sin, together with a lack of "faith," constitute the primary reasons why people are not healed of their sicknesses, in spite of intercessory prayer or other ministrations on their behalf. The well-known pioneer of religious healing practices, Francis MacNutt, in his highly influential book on healing remarks that, "the first condition, if we seek healing, is to cast out sin," and that, "what I have come to see, though, is how intimately the forgiveness of sins is connected with bodily and emotional healing. They are not separate. In fact, physical sickness is a direct sign that we are not right with God."[2] The damage that ideas of this nature must do to people in a highly vulnerable state is incalculable, and can only be described as little short of abhorrent.

The development of scientific medicine, from the eighteenth and nineteenth centuries onwards, should have made such beliefs untenable. Nonetheless, they have always existed in the popular mind, and had always been encouraged by the religious establishment. They may be understood as part of that almost inbuilt irrationality that lurks in the human psyche and paralyzes intelligence. The great majority of people are unable to confront their own limitations and need to find meanings (and someone or something to blame), however delusional these ideas may turn out to be. Consequently, instead of gradually dying out as one might have expected, these superstitions persist in what someone once described as "a foolish

---

1. Howard, "Medicine and the Bible," 509.
2. MacNutt, *Healing*, 17.

and tragic hunt for hobgoblins." Sadly, the modern healing movement, and perhaps especially its charismatic manifestations, has given a fresh boost to what can only be called a malevolent superstition.

The healing movement seems intent on perpetuating the cruel myth that illness derives directly from sin on the part of the sick person. It thus becomes possible to apportion "blame," either because the illness has been due to divine judgment on the sinner or because it is the direct result of the evil doing of the the sick person; a reason has been found and a form of moral logic has been satisfied, however deluded the end result. Thus, should one's relationship with God be damaged through sin and failure, then the way is open either for the forces of evil, that are considered to be responsible for sickness, to do their work in the individual or for God to mete out judgment on the sinner. In either case, the result is the sickness of the individual. In these circumstances, spiritual healing, brought about through faith and penitence, becomes a logical necessity, either to drive back the forces of evil and restore the individual to health or to avert any retributive action on God's part. The notion that sickness is somehow the direct result of wrong doing or the actions of a capricious and vengeful God is a malicious doctrine that has for too long been allowed to work its moral oppression. Unfortunately, its advocates are rarely condemned, and liturgies of healing continue to be linked, almost inevitably, to the requirement of penitence for some sin, known or unknown, that is assumed to be lie behind the sickness. The door is thus opened for the various forms of religious healing to enter the sick room.

THE FAITH HEALING MOVEMENTS

Since the end of the nineteenth century there has been a very substantial development of interest in what may be called "faith-cure" or "faith healing" in both Protestant and Catholic traditions. This has been true, not only of the various fringe cults, but also of the mainstream churches. An emphasis on "miraculous" healing, as a direct intervention of God in response to prayer and faith, has been the hallmark of the approaches associated with names such as J. M. Hickson, Morris Maddocks, Morton Kelsey, and Francis MacNutt. Around the world, various healing centers have grown up, in which ideas, and practices of this type have been promulgated, and claims for miraculous cures have been made consistently, as, for example, at the well-known Anglican center of the Crowhurst

Home of Healing in Sussex, England, established in the 1920s.[3] The underlying concepts seem to have been derived initially from the basic tenets of an earlier pentecostalism, and among some practitioners, a strongly sacramental emphasis has been added to the mix.

The proponents of this particular form of spiritual healing have fostered the use of prayer, the laying on of hands, together with sacramental anointing, and have supported the numerous retreat centers throughout the world previously mentioned. It has to be said, however, that some of the practices of those associated with these centers are questionable and include a variety of techniques that seem to owe more to Jungian psychology than to any genuinely Christian theological origin. One would not wish to be accused of simply using *ad hominem* arguments, but there seems little doubt that, among other things, Jung was concerned to develop a new mythology and initiate personal revitalization through contact with what he believed was a pagan and pre-Christian layer of the unconscious mind, activities hardly designed to provide Christian accreditation.[4] It is remarkable that with such a totally un-Christian philosophy, Jung has become a sort of prophet to so many in the Christian church, particularly among Roman Catholics and Anglicans. It should also be noted that the so-called "healing of memories" and similar forms of what is called "inner healing" are also based on unproven theories and dubious assumptions about repressed memories, and have little to do with orthodox Christian theology. In most cases the underlying technique is simply the use of psychotherapy, particularly thought training coupled with autosuggestion, and the whole given a Christian veneer in a religious context.

THE CHARISMATIC PHENOMENON

Since the late 1960s the whole picture of the healing movement has changed dramatically. The phenomenon of what is called "charismatic renewal" burst upon the scene and has been a major factor in bringing a fresh impetus to the faith healing movement. The development of this movement has been chronicled in depth by D. E. Harrell Jr.,[5] although his work is largely descriptive and lacks significant theological or sociological analysis. It would be true to say that virtually all communions of the Christian church have been

---

3. Bennett, *Miracle at Crowhurst*.
4. Noll, *The Jung Cult*.
5. Harrell, *All Things Are Possible*.

Healing In Practice

affected to varying degrees by this movement, with its major emphasis, not only on healing and exorcism, but on all the gifts and activities of the Holy Spirit that are mentioned in the New Testament, and that are believed to be available for Christian ministry today. The emphasis of the movement has been, almost exclusively, on the more exuberant manifestations of what is claimed to be the activity of the Holy Spirit, such as the "gift of tongues." The Alpha Course Bible studies, for example, that were developed at Holy Trinity Church, Brompton, in West London, and are now very widely used in many churches around the world, have a strongly charismatic basis and require participants specifically to pray for the "gift of tongues." There can be no doubt that the phenomenal growth of this movement has been one of the most significant happenings in the Church from the latter half of the twentieth century onwards, not least in its remarkable disregard for denominational and confessional boundaries. Indeed, this latter aspect of the phenomenon is one that should, by itself, give rise to some questioning, as the "charismatic experience" is claimed as much by borderline and heterodox sects as it is by members of orthodox Christian churches. A further reason for the movement to be viewed with caution relates to the very marked tendency for charismatics to claim detached and unique communications from the Holy Spirit. At times, these appear to be elevated to the level of a regulative principle, and any group that makes claims of this nature must be viewed with considerable suspicion.

Opinions about the movement depend very much on individual points of view, and these, in turn, tend to depend to some extent on the baggage of prejudices and presuppositions that everyone carries with them through life. From a sociological standpoint, the movement may be seen as part of the response to uncertainty that was noted earlier in this discussion. From a religious standpoint, the movement may be described as a highly individualized and subjective form of expressive religion, having a number of similarities to the older pentecostalism. The late well-known evangelical leader, John Stott, gave his verdict on the movement as "unbalanced and unhealthy," which is about as charitable as it deserves. Similar developments have occurred at intervals throughout church history, from the days of the Montanists in the second century to the Anabaptists in the sixteenth, and through the intervening years to the present; and in most cases they have illuminated the ecclesiastical sky with great brilliance for a short while, before quietly dying like an expiring meteorite. It will be interesting to see the fate of the charismatic movement over the next generation or so.

The movement has tended to foster extreme forms of healing practice, and has placed considerable emphasis on a belief in demons and the associated need for deliverance or exorcism. The specific topic of exorcism or deliverance will be discussed later, but the damage these unbalanced teachings have caused is immense: to individuals, to their families, and to church communities. One highly influential group of charismatic churches is the Vineyard Fellowship, founded originally around 1982 in the United States by John Wimber, although its influence has apparently waned considerably over the succeeding years. He advocated the need for a return to what he understood as biblical "signs and wonders," features that he believed had been the essential ingredients for success in the early days of the apostles and were just as necessary today. He believed that people cannot be brought to know God effectively without tangible evidence, and that miraculous healing and other signs and wonders would provide just this evidence that would lead to the gospel having a significant impact on society. He thus fostered what was called "power evangelism,"[6] in which "supernatural demonstrations" of God's power were to be the mark of proclaiming the gospel, and without which preaching would remain largely ineffective.

It needs to be stated, however, that any attempt to demonstrate the truth of the gospel in spectacular terms is no more than an appeal to the human desire for the strange, the inexplicable, and the wonderful, and represents a complete failure to recognize that by its very nature the gospel cannot be demonstrated in such terms. The Christian message is rooted in the scandal and the offense of a crucified Christ, and the attempts made to circumvent the reproach of the cross with triumphalist alternatives may be described simply as false gospels. There is nothing new in such attempts. G. W. H. Lampe summed up the desire for the miraculous as follows, "One of the most tiresome features of a certain kind of Christian apologetic, common in the Church from the second century onwards, is a tendency to assume that the truths of Christian doctrine may be proved by the ability of believers to perform apparently impossible feats . . . one might easily gain the impression from Bede that the evangelisation of this country (that is England) was carried out, to no small extent, by a series of conjuring tricks."[7]

The Vineyard Movement has been characterized by extreme practices, and outbreaks of hysterical behaviors such as the so-called "Toronto blessing," in which people would laugh uncontrollably, become paralyzed,

---

6. Wimber and Springer, *Power Evangelism*.
7. Lampe, "Miracles," 165.

roar like a lion, or howl like a dog. These phenomena, however, were not restricted to Vineyard churches, but were observed widely with similar hysterical manifestations being observed with the "gold teeth" phenomenon in the United States and elsewhere in various charismatic/pentecostal type churches. Abnormal behavior patterns of this nature have been frequent in the history of religion, and were common in some of the extreme sects of mediaeval Europe, such as the outbreaks of dancing mania in the Rhineland city of Metz in the fourteenth century, and the witchcraft excesses of seventeenth-century Salem, Massachusetts, as well as the similar outbreaks of abnormal behavior among the Ursuline nuns of Loudon in France around the same time. These outbreaks, however, were, and are, not restricted to religious groups and have been observed particularly among adolescent schoolgirls.[8] They represent a form of what has been called "epidemic hysteria," an emotional contagion in which shared symptoms develop in a circumscribed and often relatively socially enclosed or isolated group of people, following exposure to a common stimulus that precipitates the abnormal behavior. The behavior may be described as a collective psychosocial phenomenon and regarded as a form of somatoform illness in which signs and symptoms occur without an accompanying physical basis.[9] It seems extraordinary that such abnormal behavior could be ascribed to the work of the Holy Spirit.

One of the disturbing and dangerous aspects of the Vineyard Movement is its strong anti-intellectualism, and John Wimber was on record as insisting that "at some point critical thinking must be laid aside," hardly a biblical stance. In common with other charismatic groups, the major emphasis is on subjective experience, but with a strong emphasis on demonology and the practice of exorcism and deliverance ministry, as well as various "inner healing" techniques. In addition, all charismatic groups lay considerable emphasis on the healing of sickness as an essential component of the gospel, very much as did the earlier pentecostal movement. However, it is of some concern that this so-called "full gospel," which placed miraculous healing as a central plank of the proclamation of the Christian message, has now become incorporated into other communions of the Church, in many cases apparently as official policy. In this connection the very clear statements contained in the Church of England Report, *A Time to Heal*, published in 2000, would seem to indicate that faith healing has now been given the official blessing of

---

8. Bartholomew and Wesseley, "Protean Nature," 300–306.
9. Boss, "Epidemic Hysteria," 233–43.

the Church of England establishment.[10] This is indeed a very different situation from the sober and cautious judgments of the Archbishops' Commission Report of 1958,[11] and those set out in a joint study a year or two earlier, in which the Church of England co-operated with the medical profession, and which saw little evidence of the effectiveness of "divine healing."[12]

Healing evangelism was a major feature of pentecostal evangelism in the 1940s and 1950s, particularly in the United States, although elsewhere as well. In these years, "itinerant evangelists claiming to heal every ailment from arthritis to cancer criss-crossed the country (that is the United States) drawing huge crowds of expectant believers and curious onlookers."[13] This activity was based on an understanding of the New Testament, in particular the Synoptic Gospels and the Acts of the Apostles, that made the ministry of Jesus and the apostles set out in those books the obligatory model for church life and practice today. There was no attempt to relate the New Testament to its historical and cultural milieu, but it was simply read as being literally applicable in total to the modern world. As noted earlier, the movement also held to irrational concepts of disease causation, with diseases being ascribed to the results of individual sin (or even the sins of earlier generations) or to the influence of demons. These features have now been resurrected in the beliefs and practices of charismatic healers that are now no longer confined to marginal sects, but have become incorporated into the life and practice of nearly all Christian denominations.

It would not be too far from the mark to describe the charismatic movement as having an obsession with both healing and exorcism that betrays, not merely a complete failure of logical and rational thought, but also a gross misunderstanding of the nature of the gospel on the one hand, and a total disregard for the nature of illness on the other. It is difficult to understand how otherwise intelligent people can develop such a selective fundamentalism that seeks to import the cultural values of a distant and remote society into modern life. The term, "selective fundamentalism," is used deliberately, for it is simply not possible to live a life based in entirety on the concepts of biblical times. A totally "Bible-based" Christianity becomes incoherent in the modern world, not merely in relation to concepts such as the devil and demons, but also in respect of a range of pre-scientific

10. Church of England Review Group, *A Time to Heal*.
11. Archbishops' Commission, *Church's Ministry*.
12. British Medical Association, *Divine Healing*.
13. Numbers and Sawyer, "Medicine and Christianity," 153

Healing In Practice

ideas such as a flat earth, a three-decker universe, natural events having supernatural causation, and so forth. The various ideas all hang together as pre-scientific understandings of reality. They provided explanations that seemed to fit with observed phenomena and were acceptable at the time. Understandings of reality have moved on, however, and, as noted earlier, the "cultural schizophrenia" produced by attempting to live in a biblical world today is a very high price to pay for some sort of naive religious certainty. More importantly, however, the false hopes derived from this misapplication of Scripture are often serious in their consequences.

It was noted earlier that the proponents of faith healing frequently take the view that sickness is the result of sin on the part of the sufferer, together with the activity of Satan and his demons. Thus, it is not unusual to find that demonic influences may be invoked as the actual cause of individual sickness. When working in central Africa some years ago, one frequently came across ideas of this sort, as one does in other animistic cultures. Sickness, particularly inexplicable sickness, such as epilepsy or psychiatric illness, was understood to be the result of witchcraft, cursing, evil spirits, or other factors that may be loosely described as "spiritual." It was, and often remains, the prerogative of the shaman or witchdoctor to treat epilepsy by exorcising the evil spirits by divination or other methods, or to discover the person or people responsible for the bewitching and bring them to justice.[14] If a death had resulted, then it would often mean death for the person blamed for the sickness. Sadly, these practices still continue with little control in many African and other animistic societies and have been imported into other countries through immigration, often with tragic consequences. What is frightening, however, is to find ideas little different from these still being advocated by Christian groups in modern society, and with Christian ministers playing out the part of the shaman or witchdoctor.

IRRATIONAL CONCEPTS OF DISEASE

The assumption that illness owes its origin to spiritual forces brings with it the inevitable corollary that the approach to cure will necessarily be by spiritual means. Treatment, if one may use the word in such a context, will require prayer, the laying on of hands, and various other forms of spiritual therapy designed to restore the sick person to full health. Very often the

14. Cardozo and Patel, "Epilepsy," 488–93; Dale and Ben-Tovim, "Modern or Traditional," 187–92; Levy, "Epilepsy," 155–60.

use of sacramental anointing may be advocated, particularly in what may be termed catholic traditions, such as the Anglican and Roman Catholic churches. Should these ministrations fail to provide the required effect, then it will be all too easy to assume that the likely reasons for the failure will be either the lack of faith of the sick person or the existence of unconfessed sins.

Statements to this effect may be found in many charismatic and other writings on healing. One quotation will suffice to illustrate the underlying assumptions. John Wimber remarked that there "are many reasons why people are not healed when prayed for. Most of the reasons involve some form of sin and unbelief."[15] Such an approach to faith, so-called, is no more than a mixture of suggestibility and credulity and is certainly a total misuse of the word "faith" in any biblical sense. Furthermore, it places the whole reason for any therapeutic failure solely on the recipient of the healing procedure. In this context, one writer has remarked, "many healers exhort their patients to 'have faith' and if a cure takes place, it is ascribed to their faith. If the healer fails, the patient's lack of faith is blamed; it is not the patient's faith (properly so called), but his suggestibility which is in question."[16] The system, in fact, relies on the gullibility, and the desperation of many ordinary people who have been disillusioned by the failure of orthodox medicine to deal with their specific problems. Faith healing is thus, very often, the last resort; but it is the patient who inevitably is made to feel responsible for its failure. People are made to feel that they have insufficient faith, that there is some "blockage of sin" in their lives, that they have failed to forgive someone or another, or there is some other "spiritual" cause for the failure. All these things are directly attributable to the patient, not the healer, and it is the individual recipient of healing who is thus made to feel guilty, and often left with symptoms worse than before.

One thing is certain: the healer is most unlikely ever to accept responsibility for failure. Consequently, the situation exists in which faith healers have two great advantages over the normal medical practitioner; should treatment fail, the blame attaches to the patient and not the healer, for the healer is never wrong; and, what is more, the healer cannot be sued or prosecuted for incompetence or malpractice unless some serious consequence, such as death, follows their ministrations and a criminal case is brought to the courts.

---

15. Wimber and Springer, *Power Healing*, 164.
16. Gell, " A Philosophy of Healing," 215–19.

Healing In Practice

As was remarked earlier, the beliefs that allow such practices to continue arise from a naive, yet selective, fundamentalism. On the one hand, it understands certain parts of the Bible to be literally applicable to the modern situation, taking no account of the cultural and temporal dependence of the biblical writers, and on the other, it fails abysmally to take into account the proper principles of biblical exegesis. It has been observed that one of the odd aspects of life is that those who make the strongest claims to stand on the Bible (or stand on "the truth") frequently actually stand over it, making it say what they want it to say. The approach could be summed up in a paraphrase of the old children's chorus, "Wonderful things in the Bible I see, some put there by you and some by me!" A more humble exegesis may be more faithful to the text.

It is also worth noting that there is also a consistently strong "triumphalistic" element in charismatic theology that circumvents the "scandal of the cross," claiming that salvation means a total wholeness of body, mind, and spirit in the here and now. In some extreme elements of the charismatic movement this has been taken to mean that Christian people may not only claim healing as a direct intervention of God in their lives, but also prosperity and long life. It would not be far from the truth to say that this type of belief system is a reflection of the same approach that marked the first-century church in Corinth with which Paul had to deal so firmly. Many of its members believed that they were living a "resurrection" life in the Spirit that put them beyond the limitations of normal existence, and this sort of belief seems to be behind much of charismatic thinking.

The charismatic emphasis on what are described as signs, wonders, and miracles has brought into many mainstream churches concepts and practices which, in the past, had been very largely restricted to the fringe pentecostal sects. Perhaps the most surprising element of the whole picture is the extent to which such ideas have been accepted by many members of the clergy and laity alike with little apparent critical biblical or theological appraisal, or even with the application of a little common sense.

DEMONS EVERYWHERE

Possibly the most dangerous aspect of the charismatic focus is the preoccupation with demons and evil spirits. The belief that illness may be caused by demonic possession is irrational and is a concept that really has no place in the twenty-first century. Belief in demons is not, of course, the sole preserve of charismatic Christians, for there is a strong and, in my opinion, dangerous, emphasis on occultism in many secular films, books, and television programs in the western world. Belief in demonic possession is also still to be found as what is virtually an article of faith in some mainstream churches, and both the Roman Catholic and Anglican communions, in particular, have continued the anachronistic practice of appointing certain priests as official exorcists, with occasional disastrous results. To be fair, most official exorcists take a moderate line and will certainly try to ensure that they do not prevent proper psychiatric help reaching those who need it. On the other hand, it has to be said that the problem with most of modern "demon hunting," apart from it being carried out with an almost McCarthy-like fervor by the charismatics, is that its devotees are guided more by a fertile imagination than by common sense. The tragedies that such beliefs are responsible for producing have been well-documented, and some will be mentioned in a later chapter.

The central problem with all these beliefs, however, is that the underlying concept of demons or other spiritual entities being responsible for disease is simply not tenable, irrespective of how useful such an idea may have been in earlier times as an explanation of observed phenomena. A former professor of psychiatry and President of the Royal College of Psychiatrists, Andrew C. P. Sims, himself an evangelical Christian, has remarked that from his experience, "I can hardly think of a single case of alleged possession which could not, at the same time, and from a psychiatric perspective, be recognized as either epileptic, hysteria, schizophrenia, or, more rarely, some other diagnostic category."[17] The world has moved on from ancient concepts of causation, and the state of human knowledge today requires alternative explanations for human pathology than possession by evil spirits, even though the reality of evil itself is a constant part of human experience. Conservative and fundamentalist Christians, who consider the Scriptures to be inerrant, maintain a belief in demons simply because they believe the Bible teaches it, and therefore they must exist, an approach that one may only describe as obscurantist. Thus, because Jesus instructed his disciples to cast out demons in the first century, it is equally the responsibility of the church in the twenty-first century to do likewise. Such a fundamentalist approach to the Bible, in which it is understood as "supernaturally inspired in origin, inerrant in content, and oracular in function,"[18] raises immense hermeneutical problems with its total disregard of cultural and historical issues. There are others, however,

---

17. Sims, "Demon Possession," 168.
18. Barton, *People of the Book?* 211.

Healing In Practice

who continue to believe in demon possession without these fundamentalist presuppositions; but in either case it has to be said that those who hold such views seem to be trying to have one foot in the modern world and the other in the biblical world, a difficult, if not impossible, balancing act.

A perusal of the many books[19] produced by charismatics who dabble in exorcism and deliverance ministries, as they are also called, brings to light lists of identifying features by which the presence of demons may be determined. They are strongly reminiscent of seventeenth-century witchcraft manuals, and the lists of signs very closely mimic the features by which the witch-hunters of those days discovered the poor unfortunates who fell into their clutches. For example, those who suffer from a sulfurous halitosis as a result of gastric stasis, or some similar condition, are considered to demonstrate the presence of an indwelling evil spirit. The smell of sulphur indicates an infernal origin for their condition in the mind of the demon hunters, and is therefore clear evidence of possession. Such ideas are bizarre in the extreme, and one wonders how sensible people can believe, for example, that demons may be encountered and experienced as mythical beasts such as griffins, dragons, and the like. It certainly seems clear that their frame of reference for the interpretation of the world does not belong to any modern understandings of the universe.

The charismatic deliverer or exorcist will thus make a diagnosis of demon possession on the basis of such normal everyday human experiences as halitosis, flatulence, chest tightness, and restlessness, and the effects of demons may be seen in anything from arthritis through hay fever to masturbation. Indeed, any variety of normal human behavior, it would appear, may be put down to the activity of demonic powers. Such things as bad temper, depression, resentment, and even eating disorders, as well as more serious problems, such as drug dependence and alcoholism, are understood to have arisen in a person's life as the result of demonization or possession, for which the only answer is some form of exorcism or deliverance ministry.

Those propounding such ideas seem to be living in some sort of atavistic jungle that most people only experience in the occasional nightmare. Further, the protagonists of these ideas descend to the extremes of the ridiculous when they claim that people may be unknowingly possessed by

---

19. The list of such books is endless, and the following constitute a few examples: Subritzky, *Demons Defeated*; Hammond and Mae, *Pigs in the Parlor*; Prince, *Expelling Demons*; Peterson and Peterson, *Roaring Lion*; Whyte, *Demons and Deliverance*; Horrobin, *Healing through Deliverance*; and Wagner and Pennoyer, *Wrestling with Dark Angels*. The list is no more than representative.

demons inherited from their parents that had never been cast out. Such beliefs seem to be divorced from any normal understanding of reality, and, indeed, have nothing in common with the quite down-to-earth accounts in the Gospel narratives. When Calvin faced similar excesses in the sixteenth century he remarked scathingly, "all which they (the exorcists) babble about is a compound of ignorant and stupid falsehoods."[20] Calvin was better aware than many today that the presuppositions of different ages do not mix. The only result is confusion and incoherence.

Quite apart from the innate silliness of such characterizations, the attempt to recognize demonic signs may lead to very real dangers, particularly for those with genuine mental illness, who may thus be denied the medical treatment that they need. Schizophrenia, for example, is often taken to be evidence of demon possession by charismatic and other exorcists. Their understanding of the disease is usually woefully inadequate, and it is frequently confused with other mental illnesses. This sort of misunderstanding is frequent in popular misconceptions of schizophrenia, but it does not give one a great deal of confidence in either the understanding or discernment of those engaged in what is euphemistically called "deliverance ministry." Epilepsy has been similarly characterized as demonic in origin. More importantly, however, these exorcisms, and deliverance rituals have been shown, not merely to be useless in dealing with underlying mental pathology, producing no improvement in psychiatric symptomatology, but they have been frequently responsible for strongly negative outcomes, especially when medical treatment was excluded, and coercive forms of exorcism practiced.[21] The attempts at coercive exorcism, often violent, have not infrequently led to dire results, including the death of those considered possessed. The immense personal, and social harm that has arisen from the ministrations of exorcists in particular, as well as from charismatic healers in general, has been well-documented in various sources, and there will be some discussion of these, and related tragedies arising from so-called healing and deliverance ministry in the chapter 5. It is unfortunate, to say the least, that the numerous disasters associated with charismatic ministry seem to have had little effect on moderating the excessive claims of its ministers.

---

20. Calvin, *Institutes*, 640.
21. Pfeifer, "Belief in Demons," 247–58.

4

Assessing The Evidence

ON ONE OCCASION, KARL Popper is said to have made a remark to the effect that in politics and in medicine, he who promises too much is likely to be a quack. This judgment is nowhere more true than in relation to the claims made by the proponents of the modern healing movement. The late charismatic leader, John Wimber, once claimed that, "we see hundreds of people healed every month in Vineyard Christian Fellowship services . . . the blind see; the lame walk; the deaf hear. Cancer is disappearing!"[1] These quite extraordinary claims lack any substantiation from any unbiased and objective observers. Unfortunately, however, he has not been alone in making such claims, as a glance at many of the websites of various so-called healing ministries or the advertisements for healing services, missions, and campaigns in the press will reveal. Websites contain page after page of apparent cures as a result of mainly charismatic activities, but with no objective substantiation or independent validation of either diagnosis or cure. It is important to recognize that the validation of claims of such magnitude requires the same sort of rigorous testing procedures that would be applied to any other similar claim for a successful treatment, such as for a new therapeutic agent or surgical procedure. Merely because the alleged cures are supposedly derived from a "spiritual" source does not

---

1. Wimber and Springer, *Power Evangelism*, 55. I am given to understand that towards the end of his life, he came to modify some of his more extreme views in the light of his own terminal illness and approaching death.

obviate the necessity for proper documentation. Indeed, it may be argued that the keeping of careful records, together with objective assessments of end results, are all the more necessary as the claims for healing are usually made in the name of God. It is God's credibility that is being put on the line, and credibility itself requires to be established at two levels, that of fact, and that of interpretation.

THE NEED FOR RIGOROUS INVESTIGATION

It has been observed that the attractiveness of a belief is all too often inversely proportional to its truth.[2] There is no doubt that many people find the idea of "spiritual healing" highly attractive, and stories are told and retold to reinforce belief in its effectiveness, an example of the operation of the "Bellman fallacy" that was mentioned in an earlier chapter. It also needs to be remembered that anecdotal evidence by itself is clearly insufficient to substantiate claims for any form of therapeutic program, whether it be, for example, a new drug or a new surgical procedure. This caveat applies in exactly the same way to the far-reaching claims of the healing movement with its emphasis on divine and miraculous interventions. Further, simple observational evidence is also insufficient by itself. Evidence of this nature may nearly always be found to support any theory. The false ideas of the phlogiston theory of combustion, which ruled chemical thought in the eighteenth century until the discovery of oxygen, or the ancient Ptolemaic view of the universe, with the earth at the center around which the sun and stars revolved, seemed to be supported by good observational evidence. The fact that a certain understanding of reality may appear to agree with the observed data, however, should not be taken to indicate that there is any truth in that understanding. A good scientific theory may be refuted or falsified by observation. Repeated observations that disagree with the theory will mean that the theory will have to be abandoned or at least modified. Only when the claims in support of faith healing have survived all the best attempts to refute or falsify them, may any claims to truth (or at least an approximation to truth) be upheld.

The ongoing problem with all forms of religious healing is that, while scientific theories are open to examination and refutation, the claims of the healing movement are very rarely open to such critical analysis, and, in common with the whole gamut of fanciful ideas from homeopathy to

2. McGrath, "Doctrine," 150.

Assessing The Evidence

healing crystals, they also lack genuine logical consistency and coherence. The immense number of writings in support of spiritual healing in its varied forms all tend to be unbalanced, lacking adequate documentation, and displaying an uncritical naivete that seems to wish to believe anything in the religious domain, provided that it is sufficiently spectacular. As Martin Lloyd-Jones observed some years ago, there is a significant element in the Church that has capitulated to phenomena.[3]

In this regard, it is worth quoting at length some of the comments of a task force set up to examine the issue of faith healing as it affected the very conservative Fuller Theological Seminary in the United States some years ago. The authors of the report wrote as follows:

> Christian ministers ought always to be ready to subject any report of miraculous healing to objective, rigorous, and scientifically responsible testing. The tests should extend over an adequate period of time and be open to the critical examination of skeptics. Making claims without the controls of careful testing reduces objective credibility—especially in the eyes of the skeptics—to the level of the shaman, the magician, and the manipulator of voodoo. The credibility of Christian ministry should be several notches higher.
>
> In this vein, Christian ministers must remember that ministerial credibility is not measured by the sincerity of the credulous. The fact that many people put credence in reports of miracles does not make the reports credible. Because people believe does not mean that what they believe merits belief. Credulity arises from a deep desire that something be true. Credibility is earned by reliable and trustworthy testing.[4]

Unfortunately, such rigorous testing of the claims made for spiritual healing do not appear to have been made, nor would it appear to be the case that such testing would be generally welcomed. I am aware, for example, of only one attempt to provide some sort of objective assessment of the claims made by the late John Wimber in relation to his evangelistic and healing missions. The review was undertaken by an anthropologist who was, in general, very sympathetic to the Wimber movement. He made his judgment about events on the basis of a questionnaire given to people attending the Harrogate Mission in England in 1986.[5] Although the author did not have medical training, there appears to have been some medical input into

3. Lloyd-Jones, *Healing*, 90
4. Smedes, *Ministry*, 59.
5. Lewis, *Healing*.

his examination of the healing claims, but it is difficult to be certain of its extent. Some cases are cited in which a "cure" of organic disease may have occurred, but the only case to have been given any serious objective testing was later shown to have been very far from a "miracle," although it was presented as such in Lewis's book.[6]

It is worth giving an account of this case in detail in view of the claims that were made about it. The patient was an infant with a rare soft tissue tumor, and the whole incident illustrates the complexities and misunderstandings that may occur in such situations. The doctor who reported the case as an example of the miraculous healing of a malignant tumor was not himself personally involved in diagnosis or treatment at any stage, nor was he involved in any of the medical decision-making. He was, in fact, reporting at a distance and second hand. The tumor itself was a rare form and of a type that in about 90 percent of cases does not spread to other parts of the body. The surgeon and oncologist directly involved in clinical management consulted with other colleagues, and there was agreement that treatment should be withheld as there was very good reason to believe that the tumor would remit if left alone. The child was kept under review, and over a period of six months the growth gradually disappeared as expected. The surgeon, and the cancer specialist were both highly indignant that the recovery had been presented as "miraculous" without their consent or involvement. In reality, the tumor had simply followed the natural course that they, the treating clinicians, had been led to expect on the basis of previous experience, and to give such a natural progression the title of "miraculous" is gross exaggeration at the very least.[7]

CRITERIA FOR INVESTIGATIONS

There have been many good Christian people who have been misled by false claims similar to the previous story, and there are many others who have confidently expected miracles to happen because of such claims. Sadly, the alleged miraculous events consistently fail to stand up to rigorous investigation, and the fact that some conditions have a positive outcome while others do not is likely to have much more to do with the nature of the diseases themselves than it has to do with either the faith of the patient or the mysterious workings of Providence. What is certain is that the claims

6. Lewis, *Healing*, 221–28.
7. Lucas, *Christian Healing*, 104–5.

Assessing The Evidence

made by the healing movement do not meet the criterion of refutation mentioned earlier. The only clear beneficial results that could be detailed from the Wimber campaign related to psychological improvement. As is often the case in such situations, people felt better, their mood was better, and so on. This, as will be discussed later, is a well-documented effect of healing services as well as other forms of psychological intervention, or indeed any placebo, but it hardly represents genuine cure of disease. It certainly does not provide satisfactory evidence to support the sweeping assertions made by the charismatic healers. These claims, to say the least, can only be called gross exaggerations.

In order to determine whether cure (or healing) has actually taken place, it is necessary for certain criteria to be met. In their simplest form these may be set out as follows:

1. Firstly, any illness that is treated by some form of religious healing should not be a condition that would normally recover or improve significantly without treatment. This might be taken a step further by requiring that it should not be a condition that is known to undergo spontaneous remission in the course of its natural history.

2. Secondly, the patient should not be in receipt of medical treatment that would be expected to influence the outcome of the condition. This criterion, however, is more of an ideal and may not always be ethically acceptable. Most clinical studies of modalities such as prayer or healing touch have, of necessity, been undertaken in situations where they have been additional to the main form of medical treatment.

3. Thirdly, the diagnosis must have been properly established. This is a necessity, and the disease requires diagnosis by at least one medical practitioner, and two would be preferable.

4. Further, any claim that recovery has taken place should be properly evaluated by medical evidence using established and rigorous methods. That is to say, there should be measurable and objectively assessed end-points with meaningful patient-centered outcomes.

Apart from the International Medical Committee, associated with the famous Roman Catholic shrine at Lourdes, that is required to examine every case of supposed cure, I know of no other situation in which anything approaching the criteria outlined above are even considered, much less met. Yet the importance of requiring those involved in healing to provide a proper scientific/medical diagnosis of the conditions they meet in the course of their work, before beginning their ministrations, was emphasized as long ago as 1914, although it would seem that little, if any, attention has been paid to this important consideration in the nearly one hundred years since.[8]

When criteria like this are set down, it is not surprising that very few examples of genuine cure of disease can be found. Over the past fifty years or so at Lourdes only about eight cases of miraculous cure have been claimed officially, and they have all been open to some dispute, as will be discussed in the next chapter. Those involved in the practice of spiritual/religious healing, whether internationally known evangelists on the one hand, or the local vicar or pastor on the other, generally have little knowledge of pathology or the basis on which proper diagnoses should be made, and simply do not have normal access to medical records. They are, thus, not in a position to verify the nature of the condition for which a person is seeking help. They have to rely on the patient's story, which from ignorance, forgetfulness, or simply misunderstanding, is frequently inaccurate. I do not know of anyone involved in the ministry of healing who requires that a medical examination is undertaken before and after the healing ministrations have been performed, and none that I know of compile proper data that an independent investigator could verify.

ATTEMPTS AT CONTROLLED CLINICAL TRIALS

There have been numerous studies that have demonstrated enhanced feelings of well-being in patients with chronic or serious illness as a result of religious ministrations, but they have not demonstrated any significant effects on the actual disease processes themselves; the underlying pathology has remained unaffected.[9] Such subjective improvements may be brought about by many other methods apart from prayer, the laying on of hands, or anointing, and in no sense can such effects be seen as amounting to a cure of disease. Rather, they represent no more than an offer of comfort, with improvement in the patient's psychological state and quality of life. Important and valuable though such subjective effects may be to the individual, they represent no more than the placebo effect at best.[10] Two careful reviews of published material to the mid-1990s underlined the fact that the

8. Clerical and Medical Committee, *Spiritual Healing*.
9. Abbot et al., "Spiritual Healing," 79–89.
10. Singh and Ernst, *Trick or Treatment*, 388.

Assessing The Evidence

great majority of studies in this area were both poorly designed and poorly executed.[11] A further review of twenty-three trials published up to 1999, involving 2,774 patients, however, noted that thirteen of these trials, of what the authors called "distant healing," yielded positive results, although these results did not amount to reversal of pathological change.[12] No well-designed study has demonstrated any positive effect of religious ministrations on disease processes, only on subjective feelings. In fact, there is one published study that found a negative association with poorer outcomes in those with strong religious beliefs, compared with others, in a nine month follow-up from hospital discharge.[13]

There are, inevitably, a great many problems in designing good studies on religious healing and related methods of ministry to the sick. Spiritual or religious healing, by its very nature, has a potential to affect the sick person's quality of life beyond the primary outcome measures of cure. Any evaluation will, therefore, require the inclusion of non-specific outcomes, and will need to address as wide a variety of health and quality of life dimensions as is practicable. Although such an experimental approach will provide a full picture of any treatment effects that may be present, it will also increase the likelihood of statistically significant effects occurring by chance because of the large number of confounding variables that cannot be excluded from the study. For example, in respect of the effectiveness of prayer, it has to be recognized that, even in this modern secular age, the first thing most people do when they get very ill is to start praying and asking others to pray for them. It follows, therefore, that it would be extremely difficult to control for prayer as a therapeutic tool, making it almost impossible to undertake a controlled study on its effects.

The difficulties in designing a good study thus become virtually insurmountable when compared with standard clinical trials of drugs or other therapeutic measures. It is not surprising, therefore, that few researchers have attempted to take up the challenge, and the studies that have been published have not been noted for either their design or their execution. However, it is worth commenting on some recent attempts at quantifying the effects of intercessory prayer as examples of the general difficulties of mounting good studies in this field. The studies claiming positive results from prayer and other forms of distance healing all suffer from serious design problems that

11. Sloan, et al., "Religion," 664–67; and Boudreaux et al., "Spiritual Role," 439–54.
12. Astin et al., "Efficacy," 903–10.
13. King et al., "Effect," 1291–99.

render the results unreliable to say the least, and the few studies published before the 1980s may be completely discounted. Essentially, none of the attempts to assess the effectiveness of different forms of spiritual healing under controlled conditions have shown any conspicuous success. The only well-documented effects have been improvements in general well-being, as noted earlier, an effect that most likely represents some form of placebo effect. The strength of such effects is related to the strength of expectation,[14] and those using any form of what may be termed "alternative therapy," will be doing so as believers, expecting a positive result. However, a review of a range of alternative therapies used for the relief of chronic pain found that the evidence for any specific effect on pain relief was not convincing.[15] Even in those cases where there are positive outcomes in terms of well-being, these effects do not represent a change in the underlying pathology that could be considered a cure, although the induction of subjective feelings may be part of the reason for the popularity of alternative healing methods that frequently contain significant amounts of touch and time.

STUDIES OF PRAYER

Prayer for the sick is a universal component of all forms of religious healing, and there have been several attempts at quantifying any effects it may have on the progress of the sick person towards health. Probably the first attempt to provide a properly designed study of the effectiveness of intercessory prayer was undertaken with 393 patients at the coronary care unit of the San Francisco General Hospital in 1988. The study measured twenty-nine specific health outcomes using a three-level scoring system.[16] The author concluded that there seemed to be a positive effect, presumed beneficial, among those patients for whom prayer was offered. A criticism of this study, which also applies to most other studies of this nature, was the failure of the researchers to limit the study to specific prayers, such as those made by the friends and families of patients. This significant flaw in the study's methodology was, in fact, acknowledged by the author who admitted that, "It was assumed that some of the patients in both groups would be prayed for by people not associated with the study; this was not controlled for. Therefore, 'pure' groups were not attained in this study." In

14. Kirsch, "Specifying," 166–86.
15. Pittler and Ernst, "Complementary," 731–35.
16. Byrd, "Positive Therapeutic Effects," 826–29.

Assessing The Evidence

other words, the actual focus of the whole study, namely prayer, was "not controlled for," except that three to seven intercessors were assigned to pray daily for each patient in the study group, and none was assigned to the controls. It was thus not possible to state with confidence which prayers may have been measured, if any: not a particularly convincing result. Not only so, but the author took what has been termed a "shotgun approach" to the study, looking for a healing effect in twenty-six categories of complications from cardiac surgery. Anyone who scatters shot over such a wide area is almost bound to hit something, and it is not surprising that there were some chance statistical correlations, although the primary effect for which specific prayer was asked in the study, that is the prevention of death, showed no positive correlation whatever in this study.

Some years later, an attempt was made to replicate the findings of Byrd's earlier study under stricter experimental conditions,[17] noting that in the original research, selection was not completely blind, and participation was limited to individuals who were receptive to the idea of intercessory prayer, which immediately introduced selection bias into the study. The researchers in this later study used a different, continuous weighted scoring system that, unfortunately, shared the same major shortcoming with the earlier study, in that it was a totally unvalidated measure of the clinical outcomes. Although the researchers concluded that intercessory prayer produced a measurable improvement in the medical outcomes of critically ill patients, they were unable to document any improvement when using the scoring system of the earlier study. Further, when they applied the original scores to their data, they could not document an effect of prayer using the earlier scoring method. It seems much more probable that the results were due to the operation of chance as well as the use of the so-called "sharpshooter fallacy," that is, searching through the data until a significant effect is found and then drawing the bull's eye round it.[18] Certainly, it may be said with some confidence that neither of these studies demonstrates a genuinely effective result of intercessory prayer on clinical outcome, particularly in view of their conflicting results and the multiple end-points that would allow for chance correlations.

The third study that claimed a possible positive effect from "distant healing" was published in 1998.[19] It was a very small-scale study (only forty

---

17. Harris et al., "A Randomized, Controlled Trial," 2273–78.
18. Sloan, *Blind Faith*, 172.
19. Sicher et al., "A Randomized Double-blind Study," 356–63.

subjects) of patients suffering from advanced AIDS. The small size alone would make it very difficult to be able to establish any genuine statistically significant results. Furthermore, the study was not specifically about intercessory prayer. Both prayer and what the authors call "psychic healing" are mentioned in the the report, but prayer is not specified as being the method of healing to be tested. However, since some of the healers involved in the study were Christians and Jews, one might reasonably infer that some of the healers were using prayer in their efforts at healing someone from a distance. In addition, there appears to have been a significant procedural violation, with the protocol being changed part-way through the study. Because of the improved life expectancies with advanced therapies, the authors changed the study end-point from death to a series of multiple and indirect measures, including the need for transfusion or readmission to hospital. This enabled them to select end-points on an *ad hoc* basis, but they failed to disclose this important violation of protocol, and consequently the study is gravely flawed.

A study on the effects of intercessory prayer was reported by O'Laoire in 1997.[20] He measured the effects in terms of levels of anxiety and depression in both those actually offering daily prayers as well as the recipients. He reported benefits in both groups and found that there was some degree of statistical correlation between the levels of benefit and the belief levels in both groups. The study did not examine effects on physical pathology, but solely behavioral effects which would be likely to be affected by an individual's beliefs. This study, therefore, does not provide any evidence for the effects of intercessory prayer on distinct medical outcomes, but merely reinforces the well-established positive effects of psychosocial support on the well-being of the patient.

Three further studies have been published since the above, with considerably better design. One that was undertaken at the Mayo Clinic and published in 2001 was designed as a double-blind study.[21] It was, however, unable to demonstrate any positive effect on clinical outcomes following surgery for coronary artery disease. A total of 799 discharged coronary surgery patients were randomized into a control group, and an intercessory prayer group, the latter receiving prayer at least once a week from five intercessors assigned to each patient. The primary end-points, death, re-hospitalization, and cardiac arrest, were recorded, and after twenty-six

20. O'Laoire, "An Experimental Study," 38–53.
21. Aviles et al., "Intercessory Prayer," 1192–98.

weeks it was concluded that, "intercessory prayer had no significant effect on medical outcomes after hospitalization in a coronary care unit."

In 2005 the results of a three-year clinical trial, known as MANTRA (Monitoring and Actualization of Noetic Trainings) II were published. The study was led by a team from Duke University, which compared the effects of intercessory prayer and MIT (Music, Imagery, and Touch) therapies for 748 cardiology patients.[22] The study is generally considered to be the first large-scale clinical trial to use rigorous scientific protocols in an attempt to assess the effectiveness of intercessory prayer and other healing practices. The study found no significant positive findings, and the authors concluded that neither "prayer nor MIT therapy significantly improved clinical outcome after elective catheterization or percutaneous coronary intervention."

Possibly the best designed and most rigorous investigation of intercessory prayer to date has been the 2006 Study of the Therapeutic Effects of Intercessory Prayer (STEP) led by a Harvard University team under Herbert Benson.[23] The study used 1,802 patients at six hospitals, all of whom had received coronary artery bypass surgery. Double-blind protocols with three random groupings were used, and both the experimental and control groups were informed that they might or might not receive prayers, although only the experimental group received them. The third group was informed that they would receive prayers, which they did, and these patients were tested for possible psychosomatic effects. Unlike some other studies, an attempt was made to standardize the method of praying, which some saw as trying to apply a mechanical method to something that should be more spontaneous, and in addition, some of those who knew that they were being prayed for suffered from additional stress and anxiety that resulted in poorer outcomes than might have been expected. Analysis of the results demonstrated that major complications and thirty-day mortality did not differ significantly between any of the groups of patients.

Well-designed as the Benson study was, it suffered from the same problem that is inherent in all such studies: there is no way to control who prays for patients. Prayer is one of the first things many people do when they find out that they or a loved one is seriously ill, irrespective of religion. It would be unethical to request loved ones not to pray for a patient. Not only so, but to make such a request would immediately reveal the study group to which the patient had been assigned, and consequently, seriously

22. Krucoff et al., "Music, Imagery," 211–17.
23. Benson et al., "Study," 934–42.

compromise the study. No researcher can possibly control either the amount or the quality of prayers that will be offered by relatives, friends, and their religious leaders on behalf of the participants in their study. The issue thus arises as to whether it is genuinely possible to undertake a controlled study of intercessory prayer in a healing situation since the most important factor in the study cannot be controlled, and will always remain a potential confounding variable likely to distort the results in any clinical trial.

In considering the problems attending the design and execution of clinical trials in such a complex area, the possibility of fraud should never be forgotten. In 2001 the *Journal of Reproductive Medicine* published an experimental study by three researchers from Columbia University, which claimed that women undergoing in-vitro fertilization–embryo transfer (IVF–ET) enjoyed a success rate of resulting pregnancy after receiving prayer that was double that of the success rate of women who did not receive prayer.[24] The study received a great deal of attention, especially as it was claimed that the design had effectively eliminated bias. However, more careful examination revealed not only that the experimental procedures were flawed, but also that some of the authors themselves were frauds. One of the authors, in fact, was imprisoned for unrelated fraud, and the lead author did not even learn of the study until well after it had been completed. His name has been retracted, as well as that of Columbia University, and the study has been discredited completely. Unfortunately, however, it remains in the public domain, and is still to be found quoted by protagonists of the effectiveness of intercessory prayer.

It will have become apparent that, although none of the studies mentioned could be termed definitive, taken together they do provide an indication of whether a ministry of intercessory prayer on behalf of the sick is effective in bringing about cure of genuine physical illness. In spite of the inherent problems in undertaking these studies, there seems little doubt that good evidence for any genuine curative effect is lacking, and the benefits of prayer must be seen to reside solely in the areas of psychological and spiritual support of the sick person. Prayer may well be of great benefit to the sick person in terms of support, and general well-being, as many of us can testify personally, but it does not change the outcome of any disease process, and this is something that needs to be understood by those, clergy and lay people alike, who strongly advocate prayer for the sick. One would

---

24. Cha et al., "Does Prayer Influence," 781–87.

say to them; pray by all means, at all times and in all places, but recognize that what you are doing is supportive, not curative!

STUDIES OF HEALING TOUCH

Prayer, however, is only one of a number of measures used in spiritual healing, although undoubtedly the most often used, as well as being the almost automatic response of all those who find themselves or their loved ones to be "in trouble, sorrow, need, sickness, or any other adversity," as the *Book of Common Prayer* has it. The use of therapeutic touch or healing touch is a commonly used modality in both religious and secular situations, and one associated with anointing and the laying on of hands in religious settings, and with so-called holistic nursing in non-religious situations. Nurses have been particularly prominent in advocating this form of treatment, although evidence for its effectiveness, in anything other than pain relief, is very thin to say the least, and even in pain relief the effects appear to be largely psychological. A Cochrane Review, published in 2008,[25] examined a total of twenty-four studies involving 1,153 patients published up to that time, although unfortunately, there were only five studies dealing specifically with healing touch. The review included only those studies that were controlled or randomized clinical trials, and that included "sham" placebo, or "no treatment" controls. The conclusions of the review were guarded, the authors not committing themselves beyond a statement that therapeutic touch may have a modest effect in pain relief. A fresh look at the data presented would suggest that the effect was modest in the extreme and could be said to be minimal. Another review of studies of therapeutic touch was published some years earlier,[26] and this also found no more than very modest effects. The same conclusion was also drawn from the most recent study to hand that examined the effects of therapeutic touch on post-operative patients.[27] The authors of this study concluded that therapeutic touch may have value in reducing psychological stress, assisting the patient to relax. It may, thus, have some value in pain relief. Once again, however, it should be noted that nothing can be claimed for any of these modalities other than that they may provide some psychological support for the patient; they do

25. So et al., "Touch Therapies."
26. Peters, "Effectiveness," 52–61.
27. Coakley and Duffy, "Effect," 193–200.

not act in isolation to change any underlying disease process, and whatever benefits they may provide are solely psychological.

Although clinical trials are difficult to design and undertake, and while many of the studies are open to criticism, nonetheless it is possible to say with some degree of certainty that credible evidence for the genuine effectiveness of religious/spiritual healing in the cure of disease has not been found. The most that could be said is to record the old Scots verdict of "not proven," and even this is probably going beyond the evidence. Such a negative view, however, is a far cry from the often outrageous claims of those who are involved in the healing movement, and who continue to provide anecdotal evidence of the value of their ministries. It is necessary, therefore, to examine some of these claims and determine whether they can be substantiated. Anecdotal evidence is a poor base for proving the value of any method of treatment, and it may be said to carry the same weight of evidence as the unsolicited testimonials for cures of baldness that frequently appear in magazines and the popular press. Because these claims are often naively believed, however, it is essential that they are investigated, and this will be the subject of the next chapter.

5

INVESTIGATING FALSE CLAIMS

THE PREVIOUS CHAPTER EXAMINED the attempts that have been made through clinical trials and other means, to determine whether religious/spiritual healing was effective in the cure of disease. The limitations of the studies published thus far are freely acknowledged, but the consistently negative findings of well designed, and well undertaken clinical trials provide little confidence in the claims of those who advocate the various forms of religious healing. It is now essential to examine some of these claims in detail in order to determine whether they can be upheld. Independent investigations of healing claims have been conducted over many years, going back as far as 1914 at least. That year saw the publication of a very extensive investigation of spiritual and faith healing undertaken by a committee of clergy and doctors. It reached the conclusion that there was no evidence of the cure of physical disease by such means, although some relief of symptoms did occur as the result of what was termed "suggestion," considered by the committee to be the result of the pressures inherent in the methods used by the healers.[1] This committee also emphasized that it should be obligatory on the part of those involved in such healing practices to provide for a proper medical/scientific diagnosis before beginning any specific spiritual/religious ministration. This is something, it should be noted, that has been consistently ignored in virtually all situations of spiritual healing in the nearly one hundred years since the report was published.

1. Clerical and Medical Committee, *Spiritual Healing*.

The Healing Myth

There have been several more recent investigations of the claims made in relation to religious healing, and worthy of particular note have been those by Hugh Trowell,[2] Louis Rose,[3] William Nolen,[4] James Randi,[5] Paul Brand,[6] and Rex Gardner,[7] this latter author taking a more sympathetic view than the others. Randi, in a more general study of "fraud and fakery,"[8] noted that two basic assumptions were made by those making claims for miraculous healing. The first is that any evidence of a paradox is proof of the profundity of the phenomenon, and secondly, that it is not so much the quality of the evidence that counts, but the quantity, in other words, an expression of the old saying, "never mind the quality, feel the width!" When this type of evidence is closely examined it usually turns out to be reporting from a distance, with little or no first hand or "on the spot" investigation, or else it is a case of people seeing what they want to see in a totally uncritical manner.

An example of what can only be called a rather blinkered approach, is to be seen in the writing of Michael Green, a well-known and highly respected Anglican evangelist and teacher. In his book, *I Believe in the Holy Spirit*, he has a section dealing with the "gift of healing," and specifically refers to events that took place in East Africa and Asia in the early 1970s. He wrote of the reports from his friends who, "tell me of thousands who came, and many who were healed of blindness, cancer, lameness, and other diseases. The reality of this gift (that is, of healing) can only be doubted by those who are not prepared to examine the evidence."[9] The evidence, however, would seem to point to a reality very different from that expressed by Michael Green. The question has to be asked whether he really examined the "evidence" for the cures that were claimed to have occurred, or whether he relied merely on hearsay. A very different understanding of the same events in East Africa was provided by a missionary doctor who was actually present at the time. There was, he wrote, "tremendous popularity initially with thousands of people being attracted to the meetings, followed by

2. Trowell, *Study Notes*.
3. Rose, *Faith Healing*.
4. Nolen, *Healing*.
5. Randi, *The Faith Healers*.
6. Brand and Yancey, "A Surgeon's View," 14–21.
7. Gardner, *Healing Miracles*.
8. Randi, "The Detection," 287–90.
9. Green, *I Believe*, 177.

gradual thinning out of the attendances. When the popularity has waned, the outbreak (of healing) ends and the organizers move on to another area. My own impression is that the initial popularity of the meetings decreases as the actual results become known. I have not come across a single case of undoubted cure proved by medical examination of the clinical condition before and after the alleged healing."[10]

The validity of all the many claims of miraculous healing is open to very serious question. In general, it is rare that anyone confirms a diagnosis, long term results are not followed up, and, it also has to be said, investigation of healing claims by disinterested observers is not generally welcomed. Those medical observers who have overcome what are often serious obstacles to investigation have failed to find examples of cases that would substantiate the claims of "miraculous cure." The 1956 report of an extensive study of spiritual healing, undertaken in conjunction with clergy, and published by the British Medical Association, concluded that, "whilst patients suffering from psychogenic disorders may be 'cured' by various means of spiritual healing, just as they are by methods of suggestion and other forms of psychological treatment employed by doctors, we can find no evidence that organic diseases are cured solely by such means."[11] It is interesting to note that the unpublished report of the then Archbishop of Canterbury's Advisory Committee on Spiritual Healing came to a similar conclusion in 1928. The report stated quite baldly that, "In no case was it possible to find any evidence of any physical cure."[12] In passing, it should be observed that this unpublished report is quite distinct from the *Report on the Ministry of Healing*, published by SPCK in 1924, that arose from the concerns of the Lambeth Conference of 1920 about the ministry of healing in the Church of England. As Edmunds and Scorer have noted, the weight of the evidence suggests that the main influence of the healing movement has been what they termed, "spiritual" rather than physical, and "the substantiated favorable results are mostly *spiritual and moral*" (italics original).[13] It should be emphasized in the context of this discussion that these remarks did not arise from an *a priori* view that spiritual healing of physical disease could not take place, but simply that any evidence was lacking.

10. Wright, "A Medical View," 219.
11. British Medical Association, *Divine Healing*,15.
12. Mews, "The Revival of Spiritual Healing," 299–331.
13. Edmunds and Scorer, *Some Thoughts*, 86–87.

Published studies of alternative medicine usage have indicated that patients tend to be largely female, middle aged, and with better than average education and income. They also tend to be people involved with various causes, such as environmental and animal rescue groups, with what is loosely called "spirituality," with so-called transformational experiences, and with personal growth psychology.[14] Smart and his co-workers showed that, "significantly more patients with irritable bowel syndrome consult practitioners of alternative medicine than do patients with upper gastrointestinal disorders or Crohn's disease."[15] There is a large number of chronic disorders of this type, often described as "functional somatic syndromes," essentially psychosomatic illnesses, including such widely encountered conditions as irritable bowel syndrome, chronic fatigue syndrome, fibromyalgia, chronic whiplash, sick building syndrome, and multiple chemical sensitivities. It may be possible to trace their origin to some specific illness or trauma, but the end result is characterized by a tendency to symptoms, suffering, and disability, rather than by demonstrable tissue pathology, and, in general, these patients often feel a sense of disillusionment with orthodox medical practice, and respond poorly to orthodox therapy. They are all characterized by very strong psychosomatic elements, having explicit, and highly elaborated self-diagnoses, and their symptoms are often refractory to explanation, reassurance, and standard treatment. The patients usually believe that they have a serious abnormality, and persist in seeing it as catastrophic and disabling.

It has to be admitted that physicians tend to lose interest in these patients, and the patients themselves generally have a profound suspicion of medical expertise, and normal forms of treatment. There seems to be little doubt that in cases of this type, that are well known as attention seeking disorders, there is a very real possibility that the time given to the patient by the alternative practitioner or healer may provide the needed comfort, and reassurance allowing progress towards recovery. Many turn, therefore, to non-orthodox forms of therapy, including various forms of spiritual healing, and will often experience benefit, simply because psychosocial factors form the basis of the illness, and such disorders are amenable to what is essentially flamboyant and emotional psychotherapy. More importantly, they are also amenable to the properly controlled application of psychological medicine,

---

14. Eisenberg, et al., "Unconventional," 246–52. Eisenberg, et al.,"Trends," 1569–75. Aston, "Why patients," 1548–53.

15. Smart, et al., "Alternative Medicine," 826–28.

and the use of such forms of treatment as cognitive behavioral therapy. The fact is, however, that there will always remain a proportion of patients who will prefer non-orthodox forms of treatment, and, because of the nature of their illness, they will gain varying degrees of benefit from them.

This is also true of those suffering from terminal illnesses who feel that the medical science that initially seemed to offer so much has, in fact, provided little. Patients with chronic illnesses, such as musculoskeletal and connective tissue disorders, are also often frustrated at the lack of progress that conventional medicine seems to provide, and they too will frequently turn to the alternative practitioner. Various studies have shown that there are patterns among those who seek alternative treatments, and the patients most often using such therapy are those with chronic conditions, such as non-specific back pain, arthritis, and other difficult to treat conditions, such as health problems associated with depression and anxiety.

It has been shown on numerous occasions that this "human contact" factor has a demonstrably beneficial effect, but it is quite improper to call such an effect "healing," in the sense that it changes a pathological process that leads to cure of the disease. One of the problems of modern medical practice, particularly with the increasing pressures for so-called "measurable outcomes," has been that it has often lost its underlying commitment to the whole person, particularly in areas such as time, touch, and trust, to the ultimate detriment of the therapeutic relationship between doctor and patient.[16] Not only so, but in the modern climate of "political correctness," and increasing suspicion of the medical profession, doctors are particularly afraid of touch, because of the often serious misconstructions that are placed on such actions. In standard medical practice it has been the nurses who have taken up the value of physical touch, although often with exaggerated views of the effectiveness of something that in reality has little more value than placebo at best.

It is in this type of situation that the religious/spiritual healer will often play the role of a helping person who listens to the patient's complaints, and offers a procedure to relieve them. In the more emotional and active forms of healing, associated, for example, with the charismatic and pentecostal movements, there may be a beneficial catharsis, and as a result, hope is inspired, and demoralization combated, even though this is likely to be but temporary relief. The problem in such situations is that this form of practice, and this type of emphasis, may easily encourage quackery and fraud,

16. Fergusson, "Alternative Medicine," 26–29

as has been demonstrated only too often.[17] Temporary relief of symptoms has all too often been hailed as "cure," or even, on occasions, the signs of improvement have been faked, and afterwards quoted as evidence of something that never happened at all. The most that can be said of the ministry of religious healing is that, under certain circumstances, it may help to restore elements of mental harmony, and play a part in making people feel better by what are essentially psychotherapeutic methods.

There is no doubt that the support provided by social, and family relationships, including those coming from the often close relationships developed within a church community, can serve as a buffer, particularly in situations of stress, and in consequence provide an additional line of defense against immune system impairment. It has been shown, for example, that lower levels of social support, in the context of such frequent stressors as employment,[18] caregiving for chronically ill family members (especially those caring for the elderly with dementia)[19] problems arising from stress,[20] and loneliness were associated with poorer immune function. The value of social support cannot be over-emphasized, and it is a major factor in the value of the work of the church community. The link between strong personal relationships, and enhanced immune function is well-established, but while social support may strengthen bodily resistance, and improve immune function, it does not provide a cure of disease by itself.

EVALUATING THE EVIDENCE

The discussion of the place of religious healing thus far in this study, would indicate that there is little, if anything, that would provide a satisfactory evidence base for its value, in terms of the cure of physical disease. Rather, its effects have been shown to be limited to the provision of temporary psychological alleviation of symptoms. Verna Wright has pointed out that the claims of the healing movement in general rely on the gullibility of those who accept them without any proper critical evaluation or appraisal. The situation is exacerbated by the frequent argument that it is wrong to try to

---

17. Haider, "Divine Healing," 223.
18. Arnetz et al., "Neuroendocrine," 76–80.
19. Kiecolt-Glaser, et al., "Spousal Caregivers," 345–62.
20. Kiecolt-Glaser, et al., "Chronic Stress," 523–35.

subject what is claimed to be the work of God to such evaluation, as though the healer were in some sense infallible.[21]

Reference has already been made to the comments of Michael Green about the East African healing crusades based on hearsay evidence, and without any medical follow-up or proper critical evaluation. Much the same sort of claims were made by Bishop David Pytches some years ago, for a large charismatic crusade in England called *New Wine "90"* (he remains one of the leaders of the "New Wine" movement that has now spread through several Christian denominations in several countries). Following this crusade, he claimed to have seen evidence of the cure of such diseases as cancer, multiple sclerosis, and other serious conditions during its meetings.[22] However, when he was challenged to provide evidence to substantiate these very dramatic claims, he was unable to do so, and he fell back on the weak, essentially meaningless, and self-contradictory statement that the effects of prayer could not be measured.[23] Even the healing work of Jesus was open to refutation, and his critics were ever ready to find an excuse to call him a charlatan. The fact of the matter is that if cures are claimed, then there has to be some form of clinical evidence that they have actually happened. Should a deaf person be able to hear again, then that can be measured objectively by audiometry; similarly a blind person who claims to be able to see again may undergo visual testing to substantiate the claim, and even the claim that a tumor has regressed or gone completely can be subjected to relatively simple, and objective clinical measurements. One physician summed up the issue succinctly, "If what Bishop Pytches says is true, then some doctor somewhere must be measuring the results of the instantaneous miracles to which he refers. My problem is that I cannot find such a doctor anywhere."[24]

Others who have searched for evidence of effectiveness among the faith healers have been as equally unrewarded. For example, a mail survey of one thousand people who had claimed to have been healed at pentecostal-type services, produced only one respondent who admitted to any lasting beneficial effect.[25] Claims of spiritual healing in Canada were investigated by a

21. Wright, *The Healing Epidemic*, 220–21.
22. Pytches, "New Wine '90.'"
23. See the original report and the subsequent correspondence in *The Church Times* between 31 August and 5 October 1990.
24. May, "Correspondence."
25. Anderson, *Vision of the Disinherited*, 93.

committee in Vancouver, that consisted of medical practitioners, ministers of religion, various other academics, and a lawyer. The committee investigated the claims made for healing submitted by three hundred and fifty people who had attended meetings conducted by the charismatic leader Charles Price, a man with a large following in the United States, and who was one of the principal leaders of the so-called "Faith Movement" with its teachings, not only about healing, but also about prosperity. It was found that thirty-nine of those who claimed to have been healed had died, five had become insane, seventeen were worse, two hundred and twelve showed no change in their condition, thirty-eight continued to claim some improvement, and five were considered to be cured, although further investigation indicated that the cures were due to other factors. In the judgment of the investigating committee, none of the cases of alleged healing that they examined had actually derived any genuine physical benefit from the meetings.[26]

Louis Rose, a psychiatrist from England, has investigated literally hundreds of claims of faith healing.[27] He would send a detailed questionnaire to each of his correspondents, and then he attempted to obtain corroborating evidence from medical practitioners. He concluded his extensive investigations with the words, "I have been unsuccessful. After nearly twenty years of work I have yet to find one 'miracle cure'; and without that (or, alternatively, massive statistics which others must provide) I cannot be convinced of the efficacy of what is commonly termed faith healing."

Another extensive investigation of healing claims was made by a Minnesota surgeon, William Nolen. He undertook a detailed follow-up of alleged cures, and the all too frequent accompanying tragedies, in association with the work of several spiritual healers in the United States. In one particular instance, he was able to question and examine twenty-five cases of people who had attended a healing service conducted by Katherine Kuhlman, a well-known evangelical healer of the early 1970s. He found no case of anyone with genuine organic disease who had been helped. On the other hand, he found examples of tragic situations arising out of the unfounded claims of the healer. One case in particular stood out. A woman with cancer affecting her spine had been told to discard her brace, and run across the platform. She did so, and the following day the damaged spine collapsed, and four months later she was dead.[28] In view of her condition,

26. Anderson, *Vision of the Disinherited*, 94.
27. Rose, *Faith Healing*.
28. Nolen, *Healing*.

it is likely that she would have been dead within this time irrespective of what happened at the meeting, but the work of the so-called "healer" certainly did not help matters. Many of those who call themselves "healers," or claim the gift of "healing," are simply misguided enthusiasts, although their ministrations have been responsible for much disappointment, heartache, and depression. However, there are also those who can be described only as fraudulent deceivers, knowingly misleading, and coercing people who are vulnerable and afraid.

Of the numerous important factors that need to be taken into account in considering the issue of spiritual healing, one is the fact that patients frequently fail to understand the real nature or seriousness of their condition. Doctors are only too well aware that patients go out of their consulting rooms with muddled ideas about themselves, in spite of careful explanations. People always tend to hear what they want to hear, or what they expect to hear. Few have any real knowledge of what is going on in their bodies, and the same may be said of those who are involved in providing so-called "healing ministries." In my experience there are very few clergy or ministers who have more than the sketchiest understandings of the human body and its workings, and even less understanding of disease. Thus, they tend to ascribe to faith or to prayer a completely normal instance of natural cure. The late eminent rheumatologist, Professor Verna Wright, has given a good example of such a situation, and it is worth quoting him at length:

> "A lady from this church who suffered from abdominal pain told the church prayer group that she was going into hospital the following week for extensive surgery. Naturally they prayed for her. She came out of hospital some fourteen days later and reported to the group that the operation had revealed that the disease had entirely disappeared, and they praised the Lord for this great deliverance.
>
> "It so happened that there was a surgeon in the congregation . . . with the patient's permission he obtained the sight of the medical notes and discussed them with the surgeon who had performed the operation. He found that the surgeon had been extremely reluctant to operate and had only been persuaded to do so because of great pressure from the patient and her general practitioner. He opened the abdomen and as he anticipated he found nothing but a rather mobile colon. He therefore sewed the lady up again and her abdominal pain disappeared, but she soon began to suffer from migraine with increasing severity."[29]

29. Wright, "A Medical View," 205–6.

The differences in perspective and understanding produced two very different accounts, and very different explanations, of the same event. This is not an infrequent problem when dealing with claims for unexpected cure as a result of prayer for the sick or for what have been claimed as miracle cures.

It is well recognized, of course, that unexpected cures do take place, and probably most, if not all, medical practitioners will be able to provide examples of people who have got better against all the odds. Within a religious context, not only Christian by any means, such cures have often been attributed to the prayer made on behalf of the sick person. Similarly, there are well-authenticated cases of cures having occurred at various religious shrines, again both Christian and non-Christian, that are not easily explained in the light of present knowledge. The fact that an event is not immediately explicable, however, is an unsatisfactory basis for ascribing it to direct supernatural intervention, and explaining it as a "miracle." A much more reasonable approach to such apparently chance events is that of the Jewish scholar, Geza Vermes, who coined the phrase, "Providential Accidents," for the title of his autobiography.[30] In my view, it is a happy phrase, for it takes into account the reality that things simply happen in life, and underlines that it is not God's way either to cause them or to prevent them, but rather to use them. Most people will be able to find examples of such "accidents" in their own lives, but the fact that God may use a situation does not turn it into a miracle.

Attention is often drawn to the "cures" that take place at the Roman Catholic shrine at Lourdes as evidence of genuine miracles. One of the great advantages of the situation at Lourdes is the willingness of the Roman Catholic authorities to investigate every case of a claimed cure thoroughly. One might wish for a similar willingness among the charismatic, and other faith healers to have their claims equally rigorously investigated, but such investigations have almost universally been rejected. The original criteria that had to be satisfied for any cure to be accepted as "miraculous" date back to 1735, and were enunciated by Cardinal Lambertini (later to become Pope Benedict XIV). They were used to investigate claims for miraculous cures occurring at various shrines long before the shrine at Lourdes was instituted. Since 1954, however, claims of healing at Lourdes have been under the scrutiny of the International Medical Committee, and the members of this committee have to be satisfied that the person concerned was genuinely ill, that the diagnosis was correct, that a genuine cure has occurred,

---

30. Vermes, *Providential Accidents*.

and further, whether that cure is scientifically and medically explicable. It is worth noting, however, that the decision of the Committee does not have to be unanimous, and recognition of a miracle requires no more than two-thirds of the members giving an affirmative vote.

Much of the problem in assessing these claims lies in the fact that diagnostic accuracy has vastly improved in the past half century, as has the understanding of the natural history of many disease processes. Consequently, what might have been accepted as a cure, for example, at the beginning of the twentieth century, quite possibly would not be so understood today. A good example of this occurred when a woman who suffered from Budd–Chiari syndrome (a severe liver disorder arising from blockage of the hepatic veins) was declared to be "cured" in 1954, at a time when the natural history of the condition was inadequately understood. She subsequently relapsed and died. Such examples underline the danger of making *a priori* definitions of miracle. It is simply not good enough to invoke the use of supernatural or divine categories to explain events or situations for which no other explanation is immediately available. It is a dangerous procedure, and is nothing other than the evocation of the "God of the gaps," a deity who gets consistently edged out of affairs as research closes the gaps in knowledge that remain. Eventually, God is left with nothing else to do.

It is worth observing that the shrine at Lourdes attracts approximately four million pilgrims each year, with about 65,000 being registered as sick. However, in the more than fifty years between 1960 and the present, only four new cases of "medically inexplicable" cures have been accepted by the International Medical Committee, with a further four being recognized from earlier claims, the last occurring in 2005.[31] In all, between 1860 and 2005, there have, in fact, been only sixty-seven recognized cures.[32] Such a low success rate, as one might term it, would not fulfill the criteria for the clinical trial of a therapeutic agent; it would never get on to the market! It is also a far cry from the claims made by charismatic groups, and other faith healers, although there is no obvious reason why the quality of people's faith, regarded as the operative factor in bringing about a cure, should be different in the two situations. Further, in spite of the scrutiny of the Medical Committee, there must be some questioning, and a degree of skepticism, about the genuineness of a number of the Lourdes cures.

---

31. Dowling, "Lourdes Cures," 634–38.

32. The full list of these cures may be found at www.en.lourdes-france.org/deepen/cures-and-miracles, the official website of the *Sanctuaires Notre-Dame de Lourdes*.

The Committee has admitted "cures" of multiple sclerosis, for example, the latest occurring in 1987, although one of its criteria states explicitly that for a cure to be accepted, "the natural history of the disease precludes the possibility of spontaneous remission." Multiple sclerosis is a disease that is characterized by often lengthy periods of remission, with the patient being symptom free for long periods of time. Consequently, it is a disease that fails to meet the criteria, and should never be included among the "cures" occurring at the shrine. The acceptance of such claims means, inevitably, that other "cures" at Lourdes should also be viewed with a considerable degree of reserve. For example, the evidence would indicate that the number of "cures" claimed for cancer is not in excess of the number that would be expected from naturally occurring spontaneous remissions in the general population, that arise without religious intervention.

Although isolated examples of remarkable cures coming about through prayer or other means have been recorded, very few have been properly assessed. The British obstetrician and gynecologist, Rex Gardner, attempted to assess the evidence for such healing miracles some years ago.[33] Unfortunately his definition of "miracle" was rather loose, which tended to flaw the study, and allowed him to include some cases of healing that would have been excluded with the use of stricter criteria. Nonetheless, even allowing for the doubtful quality of some of the evidence, there are remarkably few cases of "miraculous cure" in his series, and he admitted that he had been able to find very few cases in which people seeking the cure of physical disease by prayer alone had been cured by such means. It is unfortunate that he did not provide information about how many claims had to be investigated in order to find the twenty that he considered to have been substantiated. Another physician, who took a more rigorous approach to these claims of cure, examined Gardner's series, and was able to discuss them with him. He considered that even the best case would appear to be an example of spontaneous remission.[34]

Other reviews of the evidence have come up with similar conclusions. Edmonds and Scorer reviewed the evidence as far as 1979, and there is little published data since that time to suggest that their temperate conclusions were other than correct. They wrote that healing missions, "appear to make a considerable contribution to the lifting of the sum of human suffering amongst those affected by what may be broadly termed 'psycho-somatic'

---

33. Gardner, *Healing Miracles*.
34. May, "Correspondence."

illness."[35] They went on to point out, however, that there were remarkably few cases of genuine cures of organic disease as a result of faith, apart from medical interventions. This is the real point on which all who have investigated the matter are agreed; any cases of spiritual/faith healing of organic disease are extremely rare, and, furthermore, it is extremely difficult to establish that such cures are indeed genuine beyond reasonable doubt. Not only so, but even in the few substantiated cases, there is little evidence that the healing/cure of the illness has involved other than the normal processes of bodily repair. In fact, this is little different from what is being done for much of the time in normal medical practice. The task of the medical practitioner is to encourage, by whatever means are available, the natural healing processes. It has to be recognized that diseases may resolve spontaneously, and cancers may move into periods of remarkable remission for no known reason, but such instances should not be classified as miraculous, other than as a subjective experience of the person concerned, becoming for them what might be called a means of grace. David Short has remarked, "sober and careful study shows no convincing evidence that supernatural healing of physical and mental disease is exceptionally frequent in our day."[36] One might take issue with the word "supernatural" and question whether it is necessary to qualify "frequent" with "exceptionally," but the essential point is well taken.

There is, however, a more fundamental problem with the use of such terms as "miracle" or "signs and wonders" in relation to unexpected cures or other happenings. The concept of miracle, in fact, is not a satisfactory way of attempting to explain the mechanism of events. The conception of what constitutes a miracle, in the sense of an apparently inexplicable event, is entirely relative. What may have seemed to be miraculous to our grandparents, would today be viewed as a natural, and explicable process. Similarly, what may amaze people at the beginning of the twenty-first century, may tomorrow be explained as due to natural causes. Miracle is not an answer to the "how" of an event, but rather it is a religious term that expresses the idea of purpose. It is a word that belongs to the religious category of interpretation, and not to the more prosaic world of science and medicine that seeks to explain how an event has occurred. In the modern world, both secular and religious, the word miracle is frequently used to describe any event that appears to be unexpected or remarkable, or simply something that has

---

35. Edmonds and Scorer, *Some Thoughts*, 90
36. Short, "Modern Healing Miracles," 26–27.

unusual properties. The word has been so debased that it has become almost meaningless, and the charismatic preference for terms such as "signs and wonders" is little better. In situations of disease in which a patient has experienced an unexpected cure, the word "miracle" may mean nothing more than that a remission has occurred when not anticipated, or that the patient's natural processes have dealt with a disease more quickly or more effectively than anyone thought likely or possible.

The differing interpretations of the same event derive from different frames of reference. One of the problems with the religious interpretation that consigns certain cures of disease to the category of the miraculous, whether arising from a religious shrine, the relics of a holy person, sacramental anointing, or charismatic fervor, is the underlying concept that God has interfered with the normal processes of the natural world. The cure is regarded as inexplicable, other than by some form of divine intervention. A miracle, on this understanding, is thus an anomaly, a departure from the regular events of everyday experience. But many events may be categorized as anomalies, not least the occasional remissions of cancers.

It also has to be recognized that a great deal remains unknown about the natural history of many diseases, especially conditions such as cancers. Temporary or even permanent remissions may occur in many chronic diseases, and the course of a fatal disease is rarely a simple downhill progression, but it will show a series of variations, both in the state of the patient, and the severity of symptoms. The frequency of the spontaneous regression of tumors was investigated some years ago by Everson and Cole,[37] who reviewed the world literature from 1900 to 1965, using stringent criteria for inclusion. They were able to find one hundred and seventy well-documented cases of spontaneous regression or total remission in a wide range of malignant tumors, including both neuroblastoma and malignant melanoma, tumors which, at that time, had a particularly poor prognosis. A further sixty-one cases were identified by Boyd in a review published in 1968.[38] Both these reviews were extended to 1987 by Challis and Stam,[39] who were able to identify a total of five hundred and four cases of spontaneous regression of cancers from 1900 to 1987. The real figure is almost certainly higher as many cases will go unreported, and the annual incidence of remission is probably in the order of 10/100,000 cases of cancer. The fact is

37. Everson and Cole, *Spontaneous Regression*.
38. Boyd, *Spontaneous Regression*.
39. Challis and Stam, "Spontaneous Regression."

that in all forms of disease, healing responses may be difficult to measure, diagnoses may be incorrect, even with advanced technology, and the influence of subjective mental factors, as well as individual immune responses, should never be under-estimated in the healing process. So-called miracles of healing often have very mundane explanations.

It is a dangerous policy, therefore, to use the category of explanation of an event's mechanism as the yardstick to define "miracle." A discussion of the concept of "miracle" would need a major book, and many have been written on the subject, but it may be stated that it is a totally inappropriate term to explain the mechanism of events. Rather, one should utilize the label "miracle" or "sign" as an indication of its perceived significance. Hugh Trowell, a physician who is mainly remembered for his groundbreaking work in East Africa on the deficiency disease known as kwashiorkor, and who collaborated with Denis Burkitt in demonstrating the importance of dietary fibre, put the matter well when he wrote, "certain events, set within the complex stream of happenings that constitute life for the individual and history for the group, convey a sense of wonder, of the numinous, and of the living God. These events are miracles."[40] The religious concept of "miracle" or "sign" thus becomes sustainable only when it is properly qualified, and not used of an unexplained or apparently inexplicable event, and certainly never of the non-events that litter the trail of religious "healing."

The category of "miracle" is always religious in meaning. It is that something that turns an event such as deliverance from sickness (or anything else for that matter) into what Ian Ramsey called a "disclosure situation,"[41] and this in turn gives rise to a response-in-faith to it. An unexpected or apparently remarkable cure, a deliverance from some danger, all such events may have prosaic explanations in terms of cause and effect, yet for those affected, they may become pointers to an underlying purpose and meaning in the present reality of existence, and thus be mediators of God's gracious activity in their lives. They become, in fact, what Geza Vermes called "providential accidents." At this level of religious meaning for the individual they may indeed be understood as "miracles," not in terms of divine interventions that directly rearrange the matter of human bodies, but as events or situations which give rise to a new level of discernment, and which then should lead to a new level of commitment.

---

40. Trowell, *Study Notes*, 52.
41. Ramsey, *Religious Language*, 26–28.

This chapter has looked briefly at the numerous and wide enquiries that have been made over a substantial period of time, all of which have been unable to find any convincing evidence that healing in general or miracles in particular, in the sense of direct divine cures of disease, are taking place today. The overwhelming evidence indicates that the claims of the Christian healing movement, whether charismatic, or of other forms, are, to say the least, grossly exaggerated. Some might wish to make an even harsher judgment. To accept at face value the stories of cures resulting from religious activities, however, is to share the White Queen's penchant for believing six impossible things before breakfast. There is, however, a dangerous aspect to the healing movement, of more importance than the lack of any credibility in its claims of effectiveness. The subject of so-called religious/spiritual healing cannot be left without giving some consideration to these more grave aspects, and the tragedies associated with the irresponsible, and often dangerous, activities associated particularly with the charismatic movement.

THE UNACCEPTABLE FACE OF HEALING

The dangerous, and even deadly, aspects of some healing activities may be referred to as "the unacceptable face of healing." Many medical practitioners, in both general and specialist practice, have had experience of patients who have either claimed to have been healed or have been put into dangerous and disastrous situations through the activities of those claiming to be "healers." The brief accounts that follow are representative of the many that could be told; they are no more than illustrative, and are certainly not exhaustive by any means. They do provide, however, documented evidence of the immense amount of damage, both physical and psychological, that the ministrations of some of those who claim to be healers and exorcists can produce.

It is frequently the vulnerable and despairing who seek help from healers as a last resort. Their ministrations appear to be able to provide a way out of an impasse, and the authoritative figure of the healer provides ritualized roles and actions that seem to provide support and direction when all else has failed. Those who are caught in the net are often people suffering from chronic forms of illness for which normal medicine cannot offer any real hope of a cure, particularly conditions such as arthritis, chronic skin conditions, and non-specific back pain. Others may have terminal illnesses, such as an inoperable cancer or perhaps kidney or liver failure, and they will be encouraged to believe that God can heal them miraculously. Recourse to these healers is often the action of people who will grasp at any straw that might offer help and relief. In other cases it is the gullible who have been deceived into thinking that they will find help. Yet others will have been caught up in the excesses of the charismatic movement, or their church will have developed a healing ministry which peer pressure requires them to accept, and they are thus directed to seek some form of "spiritual healing" for their illness. To decline such help would be seen as evidence of lack of faith and spiritual declension.

Occasionally situations are sufficiently bizarre or tragic to merit notice in the secular press, particularly should court action follow on the results of the attempted healing or exorcism. There have been many such reports, but the following two examples will suffice. The first example is a bizarre case that made the headlines in the New Zealand press in 2001, (reported in *The Dominion*, and other newspapers at the time)[42]. It concerned the pastor of a charismatic fellowship who was involved in the regular charismatic practice of exorcism. Unfortunately, his methods were somewhat violent to say the least, and a young woman died under his ministrations. The situation became even more bizarre when the pastor, as well as members of the congregation, initially refused to accept that the woman was dead, and then kept the dead body in the belief that God would raise her back to life. The pastor said he believed the woman would rise again one month after the day she died, saying that God had said he was just taking her to heaven to show her so she could come back and tell everyone what she has seen. The pastor was tried, convicted for manslaughter, and sentenced to six years in prison, still maintaining at his trial that God would raise the dead woman. An even more worrying aspect of this case was the fact that his church was prepared to allow him to continue in ministry, provided that he apologized and showed some remorse! This case was probably an extreme manifestation, but the violence regularly associated with charismatic exorcisms should never be underestimated, nor its dangers minimized, as has been illustrated by other cases that have been widely reported in the media over the years.

Another bizarre situation arose in November 2011. Sky News in the UK, reported on an evangelical, charismatic denomination that was claiming to cure AIDS by prayer and exorcism alone, and with a 100 per cent success rate into the bargain! This report was taken up in the London *Daily*

---

42. NZPA, "Exorcism Pastor," 3.

The Healing Myth

Mail and other newspapers on 25 November 2011.[43] It was noted that there was a strong probability that at least six people had died prematurely as a result of this church's ministry. The *Daily Mail* columnist, George Pitcher, remarked that practices of this nature were, in effect, turning Christ into a witch doctor, and he went on to point out that, "it would be wrong complacently to assume that this represents an aberration at the margins of Christian churches. There are disturbing resonances of this kind of superstitious guff in mainstream Anglican churches too."[44] This return to superstition in today's Christian churches has been consistently emphasized throughout this study. Tragedies like those reported here are likely to be repeated in the future for as long as irrational beliefs, and the practices associated with them, are maintained as a basis for pastoral ministry.

Some tragedies have been reported by the families affected by the events in the hope that others might learn from them. The parents of a diabetic child, who died as a result of treatment being withheld, provided a detailed account of the whole series of tragic events as a warning to others.[45] A faith healing evangelist had prayed over their sick child, and assured them that he was now healed. As a result the parents withheld insulin, and inevitably the child died. What followed was extraordinary on any count. The parents refused to believe that their child was truly dead, and his apparent death was a "satanic device." Consequently, they prayed fervently for their son's resurrection for over a year, genuinely believing for all this time that their son would genuinely be restored to life again. The degree of self-deception involved in this case, as in the one mentioned earlier, is quite extraordinary, and almost beyond belief. In this case, the parents were convicted of child abuse, and voluntary manslaughter. In reality, however, it may be argued with some justification, that the real culprits went scot free, and free to pursue their dangerous practices.

Professor Verna Wright was a highly respected English rheumatologist who wrote about a number of his personal experiences of the tragic outcomes of healing ministries. He recorded the sad case of a general practitioner who was a committed Christian, and who was much involved with counseling work, but who herself suffered from severe depression. This had been treated, and was well controlled on medication. Unfortunately, "she fell in with a group who majored on this miraculous healing teaching and

43. Cooper, "'We Cure HIV'"
44. Pitcher, "The Loony-tunes Church."
45. Parker, *We Let Our Son Die*.

she was informed that she had been healed. She therefore abandoned her medication, but three weeks later she hanged herself."[46]

Another of Professor Wright's cases involved a young woman who suffered from severe grand mal epilepsy, although it had been well-controlled on the appropriate medication. She became involved with a charismatic group that advocated miraculous healing through faith and prayer, and as a result she abandoned her treatment as being no longer necessary. Soon afterwards, she was traveling to a nearby town, and as she stepped off the bus, she suffered a major epileptic seizure, and fell under the wheels of an oncoming car to be killed outright. Verna Wright commented on this, and the previous case: "I put the deaths of these two useful Christians firmly and squarely at the door of those who promoted such disastrous teaching."[47]

In a discussion of the "safety" of faith healing in the medical journal, *The Lancet*, a few years ago, a British general practitioner wrote of another case of severe epilepsy. The patient was a fifty-two year old man with a history of twenty-five years of treatment and control. He stopped all medication following his supposed healing, with the result that his seizures returned, and one of them resulted in injury. His electroencephalogram was grossly abnormal, confirming the relapse of his epilepsy, and it became unsafe for him to continue in his work as a millhand driller. As the general practitioner concerned remarked, the result has been that the man, "has lost his livelihood and the firm has lost a skilled and valued employee. Furthermore, the patient blames himself for his seizures, thinking that they result from impure thoughts. Faith healing can be far from harmless."[48]

This firmly negative judgment on faith healing was made by another two doctors in the same issue of *The Lancet*, who reported the following case. In 1960, a woman, then aged 24, gave birth to her first child. Soon afterwards she became floridly psychotic with delusions, hallucinations, and thought disorders, and made little improvement on the initial psychiatric treatment in hospital. Further investigations of her condition, however, discovered that her apparent mental illness was due to a thyroid deficiency, a rare, but well-documented phenomenon, and she went on to make a full recovery on thyroid replacement therapy. She had further children, and there were no further problems until she attended a healing service at her local parish church. Following this, she ceased taking her regular doses of

46. Wright, "A Medical View," 224.
47. Ibid., 224.
48. Smith, "Safety," 621.

thyroid hormone, and her serum thyroxine levels fell to zero, and the delusions, hallucinations, and thought disorders returned. It was impossible to treat her at home, and an informal admission to a psychiatric hospital was arranged. She made a steady recovery, and had continued well for six years when the report was published, solely because of hormone replacement therapy. Reliance on faith and prayer was a recipe for disaster.[49]

It was noted earlier that people with chronic illnesses are often those who fall victim to the dangers of the healing movement, as religious healing seems to offer them a promise of relief. A young woman student suffered from insulin dependent diabetes, but was persuaded by friends to seek religious healing at the climax of a church service. She was urged to stop her insulin because she had prayed "the prayer of faith," and would thus be cured, and would no longer need medical treatment. This she did, but three days later her general practitioner was phoned with an urgent request for a visit. The general practitioner wrote, "I found her to be in a state of semi-coma and in desperate need of medication. This whole episode of 'triumphalism' in action has taken her Christian commitment many years of readjustment."[50] Serious results in similar cases of patients who had stopped or reduced their insulin dosage, replacing proven medication by prayer or faith healing, were reported by G. V. Gill and his colleagues in 1994.[51] They described four patients in particular, three of whom developed severe ketoacidosis, another developed retinopathy, and a further case demonstrated weight loss and hyperglycemia. The authors made the point that the growing numbers who turn to alternative therapies give serious cause for concern.

Some years ago, a tragic case was reported in *The Chicago Tribune* and was discussed in detail by the orthopedic and plastic surgeon, Paul Brand.[52] The father of the child in question decided to make his story public after several years of silence, as he knew personally of twelve other children who had died in similar circumstances to his own son. The child had developed influenza-like symptoms, and was taken to the parents' church for prayer. The members of the church believed that prayer and "faith" (so-called) alone were sufficient to heal any disease, and that to look elsewhere for help would be to demonstrate a lack of faith in God. The parents followed the advice they were given, and over the succeeding days they prayed faithfully

49. Coakley and McKenna, "Safety," 621.
50. Hurding, "Healing," 211.
51. Gill, et al., "Diabetes," 210–13.
52. Brand and Yancey, "A Surgeon's View," 14–21.

as the little boy's temperature climbed, prayed when they noticed that he no longer responded to sounds, and prayed even harder when he went blind. The following Sunday the pastor preached an especially rousing sermon on faith, but when the parents went into their son's room, they found him dead. They continued to pray, however, as they and the members of their church fervently believed that the power of prayer can raise the dead. An autopsy revealed that the child had died from a form of meningitis that could have been treated successfully with antibiotics had the parents sought medical help at an early stage.

There have been several other investigations of mortality and morbidity among those who rely on various forms of religious healing. There is little doubt that there is a sizable problem that affects the health and well-being of children in particular, who have no way of avoiding the dangerous choices of their parents or guardians. One example among many will suffice. A study in the United States, undertaken by the child protection group, CHILD, identified one hundred and seventy-two children who had died in situations in which parents had withheld medical care for religious reasons, occurring between 1975 and 1995. Of these, one hundred and forty had died from conditions almost certain to have been cured with standard treatment, and in the others there was a high probability that cure would have resulted from orthodox treatment.[53]

It has also been shown that those who rely solely on religious healing have significantly higher rates of maternal and perinatal mortality than other comparable groups of people. An extensive study of perinatal and maternal mortality among members of a particular church that followed faith healing practices in the United States, showed that the risks of death for mothers and babies belonging to this church far exceeded those for the State as a whole. Maternal mortality was recorded as 872/100,000 births as against 9/100,000 for the State as a whole, and perinatal mortality was 45/1000 against 18/1000. The differences are highly significant, and far beyond anything that might have occurred by chance.[54] These examples are neither isolated nor extreme. The world literature contains many other reports of the dangers of what is called "spiritual" or "faith healing," especially where it has involved children. As was remarked earlier, the practice of faith

---

53. Asser and Swan, "Child Fatalities," 625–29; also, Hickey and Lyckholm, "Child welfare," 265–76.

54. Kaunitz, et al., "Perinatal mortality," 826–31; also Spence, et al., "Faith Assembly," 180–83; and Spence and Danielson, "Faith Assembly: Follow up," 238–40.

healing is certainly very far from harmless, and may well endanger the lives of those who rely on it, quite apart from the resultant adverse effects on both mental and physical health.

It is perhaps worth recording some potentially disastrous examples that have crossed my own path at this stage, to underline that the dangers demonstrated by the previous accounts are not rarities, but almost certainly can be repeated in the clinical experience of probably the majority of doctors. These cases did not involve deaths, a matter for which one is thankful, but that was not because of the ministrations of the healers, rather it was in spite of them. One case involved a young woman who developed severe depression associated with headaches. Her church was a mainline denomination, but had been strongly influenced by the charismatic movement, and she was told that she was under demonic influence, and needed "deliverance" or "exorcism." She submitted to this procedure, but in spite of the ministrations she received, she grew steadily worse with other symptoms supervening. Fortunately, at this stage she sought medical help, and a cerebral tumor was diagnosed which, happily, was benign and operable, and she has remained in good health since surgery, although the mental and spiritual damage caused by this experience took longer to heal.

Another case involved a middle aged woman with a family, who developed a severe depressive illness. The minister of her church told her this was entirely due to spiritual causes, and could be cured by prayer, and her repentance. Fortunately, she was not sufficiently under the influence of this dangerous teaching to reject medical help. Simple investigations quickly revealed that she was suffering from a severe iron deficiency anaemia that responded to the normal form of treatment with the administration of iron. Her depression lifted as the blood picture improved. This case also illustrates, yet again, how dangerous it is for church ministers and others, with no medical knowledge, to try to diagnose and prescribe treatment for conditions of which they know nothing. It is worth reiterating that proper treatment can be given only on the basis of proper diagnosis, and few ministers of religion are equipped to make such judgments.

The charismatic pre-occupation with demons, and with exorcisms, and so-called deliverance ministry, is one of the most dangerous aspects of the healing movement. It is here, especially, where clinical ignorance can lead to disasters of major proportions. Medical colleagues have told me of examples of such disasters from their own practices, but an example from my own experience will suffice to show the perils of this type of so-called ministry. A young woman suffered from severe epilepsy that required large doses of medication to prevent major seizures. She belonged to a highly charismatic mainline church, and was convinced by the minister, and other members of the "healing team" (a misnomer if ever there was one) that prayer and exorcism of the evil spirit that was tormenting her would bring about the healing of her condition. She accepted their words, and stopped her medication following the "exorcism," and, not surprisingly, her seizures returned. In this case, it was fortunate that the young woman's mother insisted that she restart, and continue her medication as well as her medical supervision. Once she had been stabilized, she remained well on regular therapy. In spite of what had happened, her church leaders told her that she should have had the "faith" to discontinue her medical treatment. It is extremely unlikely that they would have accepted any responsibility for the inevitable disaster that would have resulted had she followed their wishes.

FAILED PROMISES

The foregoing examples are but a very few selected from the many published and unpublished cases of people whose lives have been damaged, or who have come near to disaster, as a result of the ill-considered ministrations not only of charismatic healers, but others involved in what is mis-called "the church's healing ministry." Two great dangers stand out. In the first place, the ministrations of "healing," "deliverance," or "exorcism," are being undertaken by people with no knowledge of medicine or therapeutics. They are thus not in a position to offer healing of disease, and are acting in a situation of ignorance. They may certainly seek to provide pastoral care, spiritual support, and prayers, all of which will provide spiritual and psychological benefit. But they must not be allowed to presume to offer more than this. Secondly, the whole modern preoccupation with "demons" is totally divorced from any normal understanding of reality. The protagonists of "deliverance" ministries, and the like, are returning to explanations of disease processes or other human problems, that belonged to eras in which there was no true understanding of pathology. As noted in an earlier chapter, it is a form of selective fundamentalism in which the world has been re-peopled by supernatural forces to explain even the most mundane aspects of the human condition. Exorcism has been taken uncritically out of its biblical context, and applied to a world in which disease processes have been shown to be the result of natural processes, an activity that, in real terms, is as useless as taking television sets or washing machines to St Paul's Corinth or Ephesus.

The healing ministry offers much, but delivers little. Not only does it disappoint and mislead through its frequently fraudulent claims, but also, more importantly, it has all too often been the cause of immense personal, and social harm as it preys on the gullible, the disillusioned, and the desperate, raising false hopes that can never be met. Medically treatable conditions have been mismanaged, and the preventable deaths that have occurred should raise profound concern among clergy and other church leaders. Unfortunately, little critical attention seems to have been paid to the claims of the healing movement, and its teachings have been accepted almost without question. As a result, it has come to take a prominent place in the ministry of many, if not most, churches. The examples of the "unacceptable face of healing" that I have given here are not isolated phenomena by any means; they are, in fact, the virtually inevitable result of returning to a magical approach to the cure of physical illness. Not only so, but the claims of "healing" lack any genuine credibility, and the activities of the healers are to be put into the same categories as the shamans and witchdoctors, whether they be in the form of charismatic "signs and wonders," the claimed "miracles" associated with holy relics or holy shrines, or the *ex opere operato* effects of the sacraments. It has been argued that the healing movement in general raises serious problems, but there can be no doubt that the various forms of charismatic healing in particular, raise serious ethical and moral questions that have been very largely ignored by those in responsible positions in the Christian churches. Nonetheless, these are issues that require to be addressed with urgency and objectivity by church leaders. It is surely time for an honest facing up to the issues, and an honest appraisal of both current theory, and current practice, as well as the damage wrought in the lives of so many, particularly those associated with the various schools of charismatic thought.

It has to be admitted, however, that the healing movement has become such an accepted part of modern church life that it would now be difficult to dislodge it. The reasons for this are complex, and it would need a separate study to elucidate them in detail. However, it is worth making a few passing observations on two of the possible factors that have contributed to the development of the healing movement. In each case there are features which pander to the modern search for health and fitness, that for many people seems to be almost a religion in itself.

There seems little doubt that one significant factor in recent times has been the triumphalism of charismatic and similar forms of Christianity. There is nothing new in such emphases, and Paul was in combat with them in the very early days of the faith, particularly in his letters to the Corinthians. They derive from a rejection of the scandal of the cross that lies at the heart of Christianity, and requires a life of conformity to the death of Christ with its concomitant acceptance of suffering and limitation. Instead, there is an emphasis on a triumphant life in the Spirit. Professor Morna Hooker of Cambridge put it like this, "what the Corinthians were in danger of forgetting was the implication of the manner of Christ's death for their own way of life. Experience of the resurrection had led them to suppose that the Christian life was totally positive — a matter of joy and excitement. Their experience had led them to interpret the Christian life in terms of instant blessing — instant joy, instant peace, instant salvation."[55] Such attitudes are very much part of charismatic thought, and they fit well with modern consumerism with its requirement for instant gratification of every sort. People want an instant God in the same way as they want instant coffee. The false emphases of charismatic Christianity have led to an attitude on the part of its followers that requires an instant access to every possible blessing without the inconvenience of having to pay for them. Healing thus becomes almost a right, and it is not surprising that the excesses that have been discussed earlier come into being. This form of healing ministry, although based on a totally inadequate theology, nonetheless appeals strongly to contemporary modes of thought, and such attitudes and beliefs would seem to be a major factor in the growth and popularity of the healing movement.

There also seems to be no doubt that there is also a very real sense of spiritual elitism among those who practice "healing," and so-called "deliverance" ministries. In fact, the healing movement as a whole is simply the latest in a long catalogue of such movements throughout the history of the Christian church, from the days of St Paul's Corinth, continuing through Montanism, the enthusiastic sects that blossomed at the Reformation, and the almost innumerable list of other similar movements to the present day. The badges of being counted among the elite are such things as being able to "speak in tongues," to "heal," and to "cast out demons." The practice of such forms of "ministry" provides an intensely satisfying outlet for some Christians who are perhaps unfulfilled in daily life, and need something to provide them with status, and to meet their inadequacies. Unfortunately,

---

55. Hooker, *Not Ashamed*, 14.

many mainstream churches have fallen under the spell of the charismatic movement, and encourage such unhealthy approaches, for example through the use of the Alpha study program, with its unapologetic pressure on participants to "speak in tongues."

At the other end of the spectrum it might be argued that the modern emphasis on the rather vague and nebulous varieties of religious healing, particularly those concerned with "inner healing," and similar indeterminate varieties, reflects the crisis of confidence of many of the more liberal clergy who have largely rejected a transcendent gospel, and have to look elsewhere to provide help for their parishioners. These practitioners, although not appearing to offer the charismatic short cuts to being healthy, wealthy, and wise, would seek to provide their congregations with what is, probably, no more than a different manifestation of the modern pre-occupation with the self. At the same time, however, the religious dimension of this form of healing provides a significant level of attractiveness for those who want a form of "spirituality" without the necessity of commitment to the demands of the Christian gospel, that requires its followers to live lives that are "crucified with Christ."

It has been the argument of this study that what has been called the church's healing ministry to the sick, especially as developed and practiced in charismatic churches, is inadequate, often misleading, and at times dangerous. It has simply not delivered on its promises. There is thus a very real need to give consideration to different approaches to the church's ministry to the sick, approaches that will mark a return to more biblical standards of true care and integrity. In the final chapter, therefore, I will try to outline an alternative approach, with an emphasis on the biblical understanding of the role of Christians as carers of the sick and needy, rather than as "healers."

6

CARING OR CURING?
The Church's Ministry

THIS SHORT STUDY HAD, as its starting point, the conflicting views and practices that surround what has come to be called the healing ministry of the church. It has been argued that not only does this phrase mean many different things to different people, but also that there is no commonly agreed definition of what is really meant by the term "healing," with all the inevitable confusion that such obfuscation produces. Further, it has also been shown that the claims for the various forms of religious/spiritual healing are not only grossly exaggerated, and often false, but they may also be extremely dangerous, particularly when the so-called ministries of exorcism and deliverance are being practiced. A huge edifice of muddled theology, together with highly questionable practice, has been built upon very shaky foundations. It is not surprising, therefore, that much of the present confusion about the church's role in the ministry to the sick arises from misunderstandings about what the New Testament writings can, or ever intended to, teach.

Contrary to fundamentalist, or strongly conservative viewpoints, the New Testament documents were never intended to set out a prescriptive pattern for future generations to follow slavishly. The Bible is not a modern textbook capable of giving neat answers in black and white for today's problems, and to treat it as such is to move rapidly towards narrow-minded bigotry and irrational dogmatism. Indeed, there is little evidence that the earliest first-century congregations followed anything like consistent patterns of ministry or practice or, for that matter, demonstrated anything approaching a standardized system of belief among the welter of theological opinions that were held by those who all equally held themselves to be true followers of Jesus. It was not until much later, as the creeds came to be formulated as bulwarks of orthodoxy, that some degree of uniformity of belief and practice could be imposed. It is against this background of diversity within the New Testament writings that each generation needs to find its own answers for life and practice within the Christian community. Nonetheless, many of the solutions reached by the early church, preserved in those selfsame New Testament writings, will often provide what C. S. Lewis called "signposts,"[1] pointing to underlying principles that should govern the ways in which the gospel may be expressed, and life should be lived in today's very different world.

Ultimately, the challenge is to build credible practice on the basis of credible theology, and that will not be accomplished by trying to repeat uncritically, in the twenty-first century, the activity of Jesus and the apostles in the first century, as recounted in the New Testament. The modern healing movement in the church fails to provide either credible practice or credible theology, and, as was discussed in earlier chapters, it all too often opens the doors to charges of fraud, charges that sadly, on occasions, are not difficult to sustain. The proponents of healing practices in the church might be wise to bear in mind that, as someone remarked, "to offer sick people an illusion of cure that can never be fulfilled (is) a particularly offensive form of fraud."[2]

It is necessary, therefore, to build an adequate theology for the Church's ministry to the sick that accepts the central thesis of the good news of Christ, that God is intimately involved in human suffering and limitation. The gospel does not provide a miraculous escape from the inevitable results of living in a contingent universe. Sickness, suffering, and death are part of being human, and there are no short cuts to a life free from its normal vicissitudes. Ministry to, and the spiritual care of, the sick should be a balanced ministry, and one that pays attention to three considerations.

---

1. Lewis, *Surprised by Joy*, 238.
2. Anon. "Medical Quackbuster," 1090.

UNDERSTANDING "MIRACLE"

In the first place, it is argued that a proper approach to the concept of "miracle" needs to be developed. This issue was discussed briefly at an earlier stage of the study, but the main points need to be restated. The word "miracle" is used so loosely these days that it has become almost devoid of content. The misunderstandings and misapplications of the term require that a careful reappraisal should be made of the concepts of "miracles," "wonders," and "signs." The biblical records of such events, as well as the claims down the centuries to modern times, need to be examined carefully and critically. The term "miracle" is, in my judgment, totally inappropriate as an explanation of mechanism, as was pointed out earlier. When the biblical narratives of healing events are examined, what is discovered is not some form of inexplicable, divine intervention, but an event that may be explained by the normal categories of pathology and physiology. Such events may well be labelled "signs," as the writer of the Fourth Gospel did in respect of the activity of Jesus, but such a label is indicative of significance rather than an explanation of mechanism. They were pointers to what was going on in the ministry of Jesus. They did not produce faith in the observers; in fact often the opposite. They did not provide some sort of proof of who Jesus was, a mistaken view that still persists in many minds; rather they helped people see that God was active in this man Jesus, as Nicodemus was made to say in John's story, "No one could do these signs unless God was with him" (John 3:2).

The same considerations apply to events that today are often labelled as miraculous. Indeed, very few of such reported events stand up to any level of critical scrutiny, and the fact that the evidence for miraculous healing is singularly lacking has been discussed in detail in an earlier chapter. Even those occasional apparent cures of disease that are not immediately explicable in medical terms should not be classified as miraculous in the sense of divine intervention. This is to fall into the trap of turning what are essentially time conditioned explanations into absolutes. Events that are part of everyday experience in the world of the twenty-first century would have seemed miraculous even a hundred years ago, and would have been explicable only in terms of some supernatural cause to people living in biblical times. The moment one strays into this territory, and invokes God as the immediate cause of unexplained phenomena, one inevitably finishes with a "God of the gaps" who, by definition, is a shrinking god. As the frontiers of knowledge are expanded, this sort of god eventually runs out of things to do, and ultimately becomes no longer necessary, dying the death of a thousand explanations as the gaps in knowledge are filled.

If the term is to be used at all (and in the modern world one should have serious reservations about its use) it should not be as an explanation of the mechanism of an event, but as a term that interprets what has happened in terms of its significance for the individual. Thus, an event, be it restoration to health from serious illness, or an escape from some perilous situation, may acquire a deeper spiritual significance in the experience of an individual or community, and become a mediator of God's grace and salvation. Miracle, like beauty, is something which very much lies in the eye of the beholder, and should be reserved for the realm of theological interpretation, not the explanation of mechanism. It belongs to a person's subjective experience and appreciation, and not to the objective processes that gave rise to the event. For this reason, it is suggested that a term such as "providential accident" is more theologically adequate, and more correct than the use of "miracle," or any other similar term. Until the church is prepared to accept that the concepts of "miracles, signs, and wonders" are not valid categories to explain events in the universe, the way will remain open for false claims, and continuing disillusionment. The wise remarks of Hugh Trowell, quoted at an earlier part of this study, are eminently worth repeating, "Rather is it that certain events, set within the complex stream of happenings that constitute life for the individual and history for the group, convey a sense of wonder, of the numinous, and of the living God. These events are miracles."[3] It needs to be stated that the characterization of modern religious healing in terms of the miraculous or signs and wonders is to invest the activities of those involved with a level of significance that is not merely unjustified, but is, in fact, plain silly.

GOD IS NOT ARBITRARY

The second point that a properly formulated theology of healing requires to affirm is that any ministry to the sick and dying can be undertaken only with a recognition that God does not act in an arbitrary fashion. Human experience generally, would suggest that events frequently tend to be random, and by chance. Things happen without any sense of fairness, and with the good seemingly often worse off than the bad. The universe seems often

---

3. Trowell, *Study Notes*, 52.

to be immoral as far as rewards and punishments are concerned, as W. S. Gilbert put it in *The Mikado*:

> "See how the Fates their gifts allot
> For A is happy—B is not.
> Yet B is worthy, I dare say,
> Of more prosperity than A!"

In spite of the vagaries of normal life, however, and the inevitability of chance events occurring in a contingent universe, biblical theology is consistent in emphasizing that God's love and grace are extended to all without exception, and without partiality. In a situation, for example, in which two people are suffering from the same disease, God does not decide on recovery for one, and death for the other. Death and recovery are the result of natural factors with which God does not interfere. God does not change the normal constitutive processes of nature to meet the demands of a favored few. This seems to be the teaching of the New Testament letters which provided for no expectation of "miraculous" cures when people were sick. The emphasis is rather, on a willingness to accept the common experience of humanity in daily life. St Paul, for example, rejoiced in the mercy of God when a colleague recovered from a serious illness, rather than assuming complacently that such recovery was always to be the proper expected outcome of sickness (Phil 2:27).

The New Testament emphasis is consistently on a God who is intimately involved in the human situation, however hopeless or painful it may appear; a God who is there in the "valley of the shadow of death," to be with those who trust in him, and provide the necessary grace to cope with the darkest circumstances. The triumphalist gospel of the charismatics, and those who share similar presuppositions, fails to take into account a proper understanding of the Christian doctrine of the incarnation, and a proper understanding of the realities of the human situation. In Christ, God has identified himself with sinful and suffering humanity, and the Church is now required to take that identification with the suffering of the sick, the dying, and others in need, into its own ministry as the servant community. The ministry of the Church is, in a sense, an extension of the ministry of Christ who "suffers (*sumpathēsai*) with us in our weaknesses (*astheneiais*, a word frequently used of sickness)" (Heb 4:15). It is not going beyond reasonable exegesis to make the point that, effectively, the weakness that Christ shares with us encompasses all forms of human suffering. What is referred to here is not empathy, which is no more than understanding the problems of others without entering into them. Christian theology affirms that God is in the darkest hour, and sharing it with the sufferer.

If the Christian Church is serious about its ministry to the sick, then it must be serious in its affirmation of the reality and inevitability of suffering, sickness, and death within a contingent universe that is simply as it is, and cannot be changed. At the same time, however, it must also lay equal emphasis on the reality of a God who is not merely sovereign, but also a God who suffers with his creation. The mistaken, and unbalanced theologies of those who advocate the various forms of spiritual healing fail to take these realities into account. They attempt to negate the universal experience of all human beings (and other animals too) leaving those (the majority) who fail to benefit from their ministrations, blaming themselves for their lack of "faith" or deeply hurt by an apparently capricious God, who shows arrant favoritism in his actions towards some, and not others. It was to this important issue that Hensley Henson drew attention many years ago when he wrote, "suffering saddens and perplexes, but it does not alienate us, for under the bitter covenant of pain we must all live and he suffers with us; but the partiality of favouritism, which grants exemptions from the general curse, not on any intelligible principle or in the service of any adequate case, but by mere caprice at this shrine, or at that man's hands, alarms and revolts us. Not the credit of churches, but the character of God is the issue at stake in this controversy."[4]

Christians need to understand that God is not an arbitrary meddler in the affairs of the universe, and he is not there as some sort of "Mr Fixit" to be called upon as required. David Jenkins once made the point that, a "God who uses the openness of his created universe, the openness and freedom of men and women created in his image and the mystery of his own risky and creative love to produce particular events or trends by that eventuality alone would be a meddling demigod, a moral monster and a contradiction of himself,"[5] and he went on to emphasize that God was not an arbitrary meddler nor an occasional fixer. God is not there to provide easy answers to the problems of life, and to the random events of disease, death, and disaster. What he does promise, however, is his presence in the problem, his grace, and his love. The protagonists of "healing" consistently fail to face up to these realities in the pursuit of their aims.

4. Henson, *Notes on Spiritual Healing*, 92.
5. Jenkins, *God, Miracle*, 63.

MAINTAINING THE BOUNDARIES

The third matter to which the Church should be paying proper attention in its work among the sick is the relation of its ministers (whether clergy or lay) to the work of the normal health care professions of medicine, nursing, and the various related professions, such as physiotherapy, psychology, and so forth. It needs to be affirmed by all those engaged in ministry to the sick that, of necessity, their work must be in close association with the practice of medicine, and with a proper recognition of the boundaries between different forms of ministry to the human person. Unfortunately, this has not always been the way in which the advocates of religious healing have tended to operate. It is rare to find any co-operative relationship between those involved in the practice of religious/spiritual healing, and the medical profession. They move in, and they move out, they pray, and they anoint, encouraging false hopes, and frequently acting, seemingly, without any proper supervision or accountability. As has been noted earlier, the fact of the matter is, that with very few exceptions, ministers of the church, whether ordained or lay, have no competence to assess the nature of a person's sickness, and this is something that cannot be over-emphasized. Proper and effective treatment should be based on rational, and adequate diagnosis, that is, the identification of the disease, and its underlying cause. The absence of any proper diagnosis makes nonsense of the claims of so much that passes for healing in religious circles.

THE CHURCH'S PROPER TASK

Provided that the three principles that have been outlined above are accepted as basic to any ministry to the sick, then it may be affirmed that the Christian church still has many unique opportunities for engagement with people at critical points in their lives, and be able to demonstrate the care and loving concern of God in Christ. There is no doubt that one of the principal roles for the church is to provide actively for those dimensions of life that are too frequently ignored in normal curative medicine. It has been noted at an earlier stage in this discussion that one of the problems with modern medicine is that it isolates disease into discrete phenomena that are amenable to diagnosis, and to specific therapy. In so doing, there has been a tendency to ignore the wider components of care for the whole person who has been affected by that specific pathology. Care for the sick must involve that wider set of moral obligations and opportunities that we hold towards those in any form of need, and that includes ministry to mind and spirit, as well as to the body. This aspect of care requires a high level of dynamic involvement with the sufferer, leading to genuine inter-personal relationships, the growth of proper personal encounter, and a related honest communication that should always lie at the centre of any pastoral care. True personal encounter is essential to opening up the wider dimensions of life in relation to God, which is surely the task of the church. In the situation of the sick person, this would allow for a medical "cure" to move into "salvation," as the Gospel writers would have put it, in which there is "cure of soul" as well as cure of body. It was this pattern of transformation that was a regular feature of the stories of Christ's acts of healing.

Relationships of this nature are costly. They are based not merely on empathy, but also on genuine sympathy, a mutual sharing of the pain of the situation which empathy eschews. This form of caring allows for the development of a framework within which the patient may find the presence of God within the situation, and be assured of the redemptive love of God in the most difficult of circumstances. Further, it allows people to identify the possibilities for change, and for spiritual growth in spite of their limitations, and, through prayer and the word of God, find that in Christ, he offers grace and strength to sustain and transform. It is this wider dimension that constitutes the essence of the church's ministry to the sick, and is to be seen as a vital part of that deep *caritas serviens* that was the basis of the hospitals, hospices, and houses for the sick and dying that flourished over the Christian Roman Empire, and into mediaeval Christendom, in which there was a ministry to the whole person in respect of both physical, and spiritual need.

The limitations of disease, and its associated uncertainties are part of universal experience. In this situation the church has an essential part to play, not in trying to bring about physical healing, but in awakening or strengthening faith in a loving God, and in providing the powerful support of prayer to help both patient and family come to terms with the inevitable reality of suffering, as well as the equally inevitable, and totally unavoidable, reality of death. It is argued that such a ministry is more of a practical response to the love of God, and a demonstration of Christian profession than the nurturing of false hopes by the various forms of religious healing. Further, such a ministry works beside, and is supportive of, the work of curative medicine. It does not attempt to usurp the prerogatives and functions of those disciplines that seek to apply scientific knowledge to the correct treatment of human pathology, nor does it attempt to provide its own diagnosis of disease conditions based on its own metaphysical presuppositions, and engage in forms of magic in which the aim is to coerce God, and exploit his power in order to try and make him serve our own human purposes for personal benefit and gain. A proper ministry to the sick and dying will work beside the medical professions as an active partner, so that together they may give a true service to the whole person. The church's ministry in caring for the sick, therefore, is to be seen as complementary to medicine in the true sense, and can never be an alternative.

It would thus be better, in one sense, not to speak of the church's ministry of healing at all. There is a sense in which the therapeutic model may be applied to much of the church's mission in the world, although it is not a dominant model in the New Testament, figuring much more in the writings of the early Church Fathers. The church should be a community of care, through which the love and forgiveness of God in Christ is mediated to the world. While all may not need "cure," there can be no doubt that in this broader sense of the "cure of souls," all need healing in terms of their relationship to God. The Scottish theologian, J. S. Stewart, once remarked that, "wherever the church truly proclaims the forgiveness of sins there the healing ministry is veritably at work."[6]

Ministry to the sick should not, therefore, be considered as something set apart, and different in kind from other forms of ministry. It may be developed differently, just as there will be differences between a ministry to the elderly, and a ministry to youth, but the word of the gospel is to all people, everywhere. A true ministry of healing is engagement in the task of proclaiming the word of forgiveness and reconciliation, the task of calling people to commitment, and the obedience of faith, so that they may become disciples of Christ, experience the forgiveness of sins, the new life of the Spirit of God, and be incorporated by baptism into the community of faith.

How then may a ministry to the sick be developed, having at its base the concept of care and not cure? If it is to be part of the total ministry of the good news of Christ, then its form should be bounded by the parameters that delineate the functions of the church as continuing the mediation of God's loving concern in Christ to the world. As with any form of ministry, there is a need for balance, and the development of a harmony between the largely (but not exclusively) physical aspects of medical cure, and what may be termed the psycho-spiritual aspects of the church's contribution to

6. Stewart, *A Faith to Proclaim*, 50.

the sick person's welfare. It is the lack of balance which is one of the great problems with much of the practical expressions of the healing movement. John Stott was on record as remarking that the charismatic movement is both "unbalanced and unhealthy," and these features are certainly evident in its approach to the practice of healing. The need is, thus, for an ongoing and fruitful development of useful co-operation between doctors and pastors in the service of people in need, recognizing that such service can only be truly effective when both hold firmly to their own well-established disciplines and to their areas of competence.

In many countries, within the hospital situation, as well as in care centers, homes, and hospitals for the elderly, there has been recognition of the spiritual needs of patients and residents, and official chaplains work closely with medical and other staff, providing for the total care of the person. Outside the hospital situation, however, the situation is less well-defined, although in some countries the groundwork for such co-operative ventures between doctors and clergy has been laid down. In the United Kingdom, for example, a report of the Joint Working Party of the Royal College of General Practitioners and the Churches' Council for Health and Healing[7] recommended the encouragement of, "closer cooperation between general practitioners and ministers of religion in the day-to-day care of patients." There have been several informal ventures, but few formal ones. An exception to the general rule was the development of the St Marylebone Healing and Counseling Centre in London, England. This center has changed its form and practice, and to some extent its philosophy, over the years since its inception, but it began as an attempt to unite a National Health Service general practice unit with the work of the church on the premises of St Marylebone Parish Church in North London.[8]

Some years ago, I had the privilege of visiting this center not long after its inception. The stated aim was to bring church and general practice together, not so much by attaching a chaplain to a general practice (an idea that does not seem ever to have been tried formally) but by integrating the distinct and separate ministries of church and medicine for the benefit of the whole person. The two areas of function were to remain separate, but complement each other in practice. It was thus possible to visit

---

7. Churches' Council for Health and Healing/Royal College of General Practitioners, *Whole Person Medicine*. See also Jones, "A Survey," 280–83.

8. The underlying philosophy and the work of this center has been discussed in Hamel-Cooke and Cope, "Not an Alternative," 1934–36, and by McLaren, *Professions*.

the doctor without seeing the priest, and it was possible to visit the priest without consulting the doctor, but all who used the center knew that the option of being referred by either to the other was always open to them should they so wish. The approach was designed to be multidisciplinary, because treatment and ministry were seen as belonging together, and all the carers, medical and religious, were involved in clinical meetings and case discussions. There have been changes in both the underlying philosophy, as well as in the practice at the centre, that have developed in the intervening years since it was established in the 1980s, and one would have reservations about the way in which things have developed under the differing outlook and individual philosophies of a changing management. There can be little doubt that it has moved away significantly from the founding principles set out by Hamel-Cooke and Cope in 1983. Nonetheless, the original pattern has provided an example of an innovative, indeed one might say almost a courageous, approach to meeting the need for active and effective cooperation between doctors and clergy, in which there is a recognition of the pathological basis of illness, and, at the same time, the need to minister to those deeper spiritual needs of the person that pathological processes may so readily disturb. It is perhaps, a reflection of entrenched attitudes, and professional suspicions that, to my knowledge, this experiment has not been repeated elsewhere.

In conclusion, one final thought may be offered. The essential function of the Christian church is to point to Christ, and to call people to follow him. It exists for no other purpose, as Lesslie Newbigin once put it, "The church exists to testify that there is someone, that he has spoken, and that we can begin to know his purpose and to direct our personal and public lives by it."[9] The church to be the church, the community of the people of God, must be the missionary church, but unfortunately, in common with many organizations, it has all too often found it more attractive to try to operate outside the parameters of its defined tasks, and to adopt practices that, in trying to be all things to all people, finish by being nothing to anybody. The area of healing is one such example, and the modern healing movement, particularly in its charismatic forms, has been associated with false expectations, misguided activity, spiritual disillusionment, and innumerable personal and family tragedies. Through its failure to recognize its proper commission, as well as the boundaries of its competence, the church has consistently encouraged, if not actively, at least by default, the growth of

9. Newbigin, *Foolishness to the Greeks*, 94.

the wide variety of strange, and often dangerous practices, made by people without qualifications or commission. It was noted at an earlier stage of this study that any effective therapy is dependent on rational and adequate diagnosis, and it is the absence of these essential features in dealing with sickness that make nonsense of so much of what passes for healing in the healing ministry. As Turner noted, the "effective management of illness or disability has to be based on the identification of the underlying cause, i.e. adequate diagnosis, and not simply on relief of symptoms which is often, mistakenly, regarded as 'healing'."[10]

Church leaders need to turn their back on such practices, and have the courage to denounce them. Instead of the false hopes engendered by the healing movement, the church needs to bring genuine care at all stages of life, to be prepared to give practical, and firm moral guidance on such issues as those surrounding conception, pregnancy, and birth, to provide genuine care for the sick and suffering, to give companionship to the lonely, and to offer the peace, love, and forgiveness of God to the dying. In short, it needs to recapture the essence of the gospel of God's grace, sufficient for all in all situations, and to put into practice once again the words of Paul, "Blessed be the God and Father of our Lord Jesus Christ, the Father of mercies and the God of all consolation, who consoles us in all our affliction so that we may be able to console those who are in any affliction with the consolation with which we ourselves are consoled by God" (2 Cor 1:3–5).

As I remarked earlier, such activity is costly for it will involve a mutual sharing of the pain of the situations encountered, but it is a reflection of the ministry of Christ that we are called upon to imitate. There are no short cuts. The gospel story of the temptation of Jesus in the desert emphasizes just this point. Jesus had to face the decision of how he was to accomplish his mission of revealing God's rule to his contemporaries. Was it to be the path of self-assertiveness or of self-sacrifice, the path of show or of quiet perseverance, the way of domination or of service? The gospel story makes it clear that he deliberately rejected the path of power and glory, or of seducing the people by miracle and wonder, and chose the way of God through humility and pain. He was to emphasize this in his emphatic rejection of a plea from the religious establishment for a sign, castigating them as an "evil and adulterous generation" for asking for signs (Matt 12:39). The message of Jesus does not try to remove what cannot be removed. Pain and sickness are normal, not abnormal, elements of human experience, and the realities

10   Turner, "Healing."

of suffering, sickness, and ultimately death, are all unavoidable parts of being human, from which the Christian gospel gives no immunity. It is only through a ministry of true care, and compassionate service that recognizes and accepts these realities, that a genuine framework can be built which will enable the sick to live to the fullest extent within the inevitable limitations of their sickness, and will allow them to experience the reality of God's love and grace in the most difficult of circumstances. In so doing, it will help to bring about the only form of "healing" that the church is competent to bring, namely that profound healing of the fundamental "dis-ease" that afflicts all humanity, and arises from our fractured relationships with God. It is this that lies at the heart of the Christian gospel, and the church needs to recover its true task, and its genuine reason for existence, in proclaiming that gospel as a powerful summons to men and women to submit their lives to the rule of the living God, thus transforming human character, motivation, and behavior, and bringing forth the true marks of God's kingdom in faith, hope, and love.

BIBLIOGRAPHY

Abbot, N. C. et al. "Spiritual Healing as a Therapy for Chronic Pain: A Randomized Clinical Trial." *Pain* 91 (2001) 79–89.
Anderson, Robert Mapes. *Vision of the Disinherited: The Making of American Pentecostalism*. New York: Oxford University Press, 1979.
Anonymous. "Editorial." *Journal of the American Medical Association* 280 (1998) 1618–19.
Anonymous. "Notes and News: Medical Quackbuster." *Lancet* i (1989) 1090.
Archbishops' Commission. *Church's Ministry of Healing*. London: Church House, 1958.
Arnetz, Bengt B. et al. "Neuroendocrine and Immunologic Effects of Unemployment and Job Insecurity." *Psychotherapy and Psychosomatics* 55 (1991) 76–80
Asser, Seth M., and Rita Swan. "Child Fatalities from Religion-motivated Medical Neglect." *Pediatrics* 101 (1998) 625–29.
Astin, John A. "Why Patients Use Alternative Medicine: Results of a National Survey." *Journal of the American Medical Association* 279 (1998) 1548–53.
——— et al. "The Efficacy of 'Distant Healing': A Systematic Review of Randomized Trials." *Annals of Internal Medicine* 132 (2000) 903–10.
——— et al. "Intercessory Prayer and Cardiovascular Disease Progression in a Coronary Care Unit Population: A Randomized Controlled Trial." *Mayo Clinic Proceedings* 76 (2001) 1192–98.
Bartholomew, Robert E., and Simon Wesseley. "Protean Nature of Mass Sociogenic Illness: From Possessed Nuns to Chemical and Biological Terrorism Fears." *British Journal of Psychiatry* 180 (2002) 300–306.
Barton, John. *People of the Book? The Authority of the Bible in Christianity*. London: SPCK, 1988.
Bennett, George. *Miracle at Crowhurst*. Evesham, UK: James, 1970.
Benson, Herbert et al. "Study of the Therapeutic Effects of Intercessory Prayer (STEP) in Cardiac Bypass Patients: A Multicenter Randomized Trial of Uncertainty and Certainty of Receiving Intercessory Prayer." *American Heart Journal* 151 (2006) 934–42.
Board of Science and Education. *Alternative Therapies*. London: British Medical Association, 1987.
Boss, Leslie P. "Epidemic Hysteria: A Review of the Published Literature." *Epidemiologic Re-views* 19 (1997) 233–43.
Boudreaux, Edwin D. et al. "Spiritual Role in Healing: An Alternative Way of Thinking." *Primary Care* 29 (2002) 439–54.

Bibliography

Boyd, William. *The Spontaneous Regression of Cancer*. Springfield, IL: Thomas, 1966.

Brand, Paul, with Philip Yancey. "A Surgeon's View of Divine Healing." *Christianity Today* 27 (18) (1983) 14–21.

Briskman, Larry. "Doctors and Witchdoctors: Which Doctors Are Which?" *British Medical Journal* 295 (1987) 1108–10.

British Medical Association. *Divine Healing and Co-operation between Doctors and Clergy*. London: British Medical Association, 1956.

Brody, Howard, and Franklin G. Miller. "Lessons from Recent Research about the Placebo Effect—From Art to Science." *Journal of the American Medical Association* 306 (2011) 2612–13.

Byrd, Randolph C. "Positive Therapeutic Effects of Intercessory Prayer in a Coronary Care Unit Population." *Southern Medical Journal* 81/7 (1988) 826–29.

Calvin, John. *The Institutes of the Christian Religion*. Vol. 2. London: James Clarke, 1949.

Cardozo, L. J., and M. G. Patel. "Epilepsy in Zambia." *East African Medical Journal* 53 (1976) 488–93.

Carroll, Lewis. *Alice's Adventures in Wonderland*. London: Pan, 1947 (orig. 1865).

———. *Through the Looking Glass and What Alice Found There*. London: Pan, 1947 (orig. 1871).

———. *The Hunting of the Snark: An Agony in Eight Fits*. Online: http://ebooks.adelaide.edu.au/c/carroll/lewis/index.html (orig. 1876).

Cha, K. Y. et al. "Does Prayer Influence the Success of In Vitro Fertilization–Embryo Transfer? Report of a Masked, Randomized Trial." *Journal of Reproductive Medicine* 46/9 (2001) 781–87.

Challis, G. B., and H. J. Stam. "The Spontaneous Regression of Cancer: A Review of Cases from 1900 to 1987." *Acta Oncologica* 29 (1990) 545–50.

Church of England Review Group. *A Time to Heal: A Contribution towards the Ministry of Healing*. London: Church House, 2000.

Churches' Council for Health and Healing/Royal College of General Practitioners. *Whole Person Medicine: A Christian Perspective*. London: CCHH, 1989.

Clerical and Medical Committee of Inquiry. *Spiritual Healing: Report of a Clerical and Medical Committee of Inquiry into Spiritual, Faith and Mental Healing*. London: Macmillan, 1914.

Coakley, Amanda Bulette, and M. E. Duffy. "The Effect of Therapeutic Touch on Postoperative Patients." *Journal of Holistic Nursing* 28/3 (2010) 193–200.

Coakley, D. V., and G. W. McKenna. "Safety of Faith Healing." *Lancet* i (1986) 621.

Cooper, Rob. "We Cure HIV with Anointing Water." *Daily Mail* (London) 25 November 2011. Online: http://dailymail.co.uk/news/article-2066106.

Dale, J. R., and D. I. Ben-Tovim. "Modern or Traditional: A Study of Treatment Preferences for Neuropsychiatric Patients in Botswana." *British Journal of Psychiatry* 145 (1984) 187–92.

Department for Work and Pensions (UK). *Cohort Estimates of Life Expectancy at Age 65*. DWP: London, 2011.

———. *Number of Future Centenarians by Age Group*. DWP: London, 2011.

Dowling, StJ. "Lourdes Cures and Their Medical Assessment." *Journal of the Royal Society of Medicine* 77 (1984) 634–38.

Dunn, James G. D. *Jesus and the Spirit*. London: SCM, 1975.

Edmunds, Vincent, and Gordon Scorer, editors. *Some Thoughts on Faith Healing*. 3rd ed. London: Christian Medical Fellowship, 1979.

Bibliography

Eisenberg, David M. et al. "Unconventional Medicine in the United States." *New England Journal of Medicine* 328 (1993) 246–52.

——— et al. "Trends in CAM Use in the United States: 1990–1997. Results of a Follow-up National Survey." *Journal of the American Medical Association* 280 (1998) 1569–1575.

Ernst, Edzard. "Complementary Medicine: Too Good to Be True?" *Journal of the Royal Society of Medicine* 92 (1999) 1–2.

Everson, Tilden C., and Warren H. Cole. *Spontaneous Regression of Cancer*. Philadelphia: Saunders, 1966.

Fergusson, A. "Alternative Medicine: A Review." *Journal of the Christian Medical Fellowship* 34 (2) (1988) 26–29.

Ferngren, Gary B. "Early Christianity as a Religion of Healing." *Bulletin of the History of Medicine* 66 (1992) 1–15.

Finniss, Damien G., et al. "Biological, Clinical, and Ethical Advances of Placebo Effects." *Lancet* 375 (2010) 686–95.

Fox, R. "Healing Powers." *Journal of the Royal Society of Medicine* 91 (1998) 177.

Francis, Leslie J., and Jeff Astley, editors. *Psychological Perspectives on Prayer*. Leominster, UK: Gracewing, 2000.

Gardner, Rex. *Healing Miracles: A Doctor Investigates*. London: Darton, Longman & Todd, 1986.

Gell, C. W. M. "A Philosophy of Healing: Miraculous Cures and the Nature of Health." *London Quarterly and Holborn Review* 178 (1953) 215–19.

Gill, G. V., et al. "Diabetes and Alternative Medicine: Cause for Concern." *Diabetic Medicine* 11 (1994) 210–13.

Glik, Deborah C. "Psychosocial Wellness among Spiritual Healing Participants." *Social Science and Medicine* 22 (1986) 579–86.

Green, Michael. *I Believe in the Holy Spirit*. London: Hodder & Stoughton, 1979.

Greenwood, W. A. "Leprosy." *The Bible Educator* 4 (1876) 76–78.

Gusmer, Charles W. *The Ministry of Healing in the Church of England: An Ecumenical Liturgical Study*. Great Wakering, UK: Mayhew-McCrimmon, 1974.

Haider, S. L. "Divine Healing." *Journal of the Royal College of General Practitioners* 36 (1986) 223.

Hamel-Cooke, C. K., and D. H. P. Cope. "Not an Alternative Medicine at St Marylebone Parish Church." *British Medical Journal* 287 (1983) 1934–36.

Hammond, Frank, and Ida Mae. *Pigs in the Parlor: A Practical Guide to Deliverance*. Kirkwood, MO: Impact Books, 1973.

Harrell, David Edwin Jr. *All Things Are Possible: The Healing and Charismatic Revivals in Modern America*. Bloomington: Indiana University Press, 1976.

Harris, W. S., et al. "A Randomized, Controlled Trial of the Effects of Remote, Intercessory Prayer on Outcomes in Patients Admitted to the Coronary Care Unit." *Archives of Internal Medicine* 159/19 (1999) 2273–78.

Hawking, Stephen W. *A Brief History of Time: From the Big Bang to Black Holes*. London: Bantam Books, 1989.

Helman, Cecil G. "Limits of Biomedical Explanation." *Lancet* 337 (1991) 1080–83.

Henson, H. Hensley. *Notes on Spiritual Healing*. London: Williams & Norgate, 1925. Quoted in *Some Thoughts on Faith Healing*, edited by Vincent Edmonds, and G. Scorer, 92. 3rd ed. London: Christian Medical Fellowship, 1979.

Bibliography

Hexham, I. "Some Aspects of Religion and Spiritual Healing in Cultsville, a Contemporary American City." In *The Church and Healing*, edited by W. J. Shiell, 415–29. Studies in Church History 19. Oxford: Blackwell, 1982.

Hickey, K. S., and L. Lyckholm. "Child Welfare versus Parental Autonomy: Medical Ethics, the Law, and Faith-based Healing." *Theoretical Medicine and Bioethics* 25 (2004) 265–76.

Hooker, Morna D. *Not Ashamed of the Gospel: New Testament Interpretations of the Death of Christ*. Carlisle, UK: Paternoster, 1994.

Horrobin, Peter J. *Healing through Deliverance: The Biblical Basis*. Chichester, UK: Sovereign World, 1991.

Howard, J. Keir. "Metals and Man: How Real Are the Risks?" *Proceedings of the Royal Society of New Zealand* 15 (1985) 403–10.

———. "Chemical residues in food: a perspective on hazard and risk." *Proceedings of the Nutrition Society of New Zealand* 13 (1988) 27–33.

———. "Medicine and the Bible." In *The Oxford Companion to the Bible*, edited by B. M. Metzger, and M. Coggan, 509. New York: Oxford University Press, 1993.

———. *Disease and Healing in the New Testament: An Analysis and Interpretation*. Lanham, MD: University Press of America, 2001.

———. *Medicine, Miracle and Myth in the New Testament*. Eugene, OR: Resource Publications, 2010.

Hurding, R. F. "Healing." In *Medicine and the Bible*, edited by Bernard Palmer, 191–216. Exeter, UK: Paternoster, 1986.

Jenkins, David E. *God, Miracle and the Church of England*. London: SCM, 1987.

Jones, A. W. "A Survey of General Practitioner Attitudes to the Involvement of Clergy in Patient Care." *British Journal of General Practice* 40 (1990) 280–83.

Kaptchuk, T. J. "The Placebo Effect in Alternative Medicine: Can the Performance of a Healing Ritual Have Clinical Significance?" *Annals of Internal Medicine* 136 (2002) 817–25.

Kaunitz, A. M., et al. "Perinatal and Maternal Mortality in a Group Avoiding Obstetric Care." *American Journal of Obstetrics and Gynecology* 150 (1984) 826–31.

Kiecolt-Glaser, J. K., et al. "Chronic Stress and Immunity in Family Care-givers for Alzheimer's Disease Victims." *Psychosomatic Medicine* 49 (1987) 523–35.

——— et al. "Spousal Caregivers of Dementia Victims: Longitudinal Changes in Immunity and Health." *Psychosomatic Medicine* 53 (1991) 345–62.

——— et al. "Psychoneuroimmunology and Psychosomatic Medicine: Back to the Future." *Psychosomatic Medicine* 64 (2002) 15–28.

King, M. et al. "The Effect of Religious Belief on Outcome from Illness." *Social Science and Medicine* 48 (1999) 1291–1299.

Kirsch, I. "Specifying Nonspecifics: Psychological Mechanisms of Placebo Effects." In *The Placebo Effect: Interdisciplinary Explorations*, edited by A. Harrington, 166–86. Cambridge: Harvard University Press, 1997.

Krucoff, M. W., et al. "Music, Imagery, Touch, and Prayer as Adjuncts to Interventional Cardiac Care: The Monitoring and Actualisation of Noetic Trainings (MANTRA) II Randomised Study." *Lancet* 366 (2005) 211–17.

Lampe, G. W. H. "Miracles in the Acts of the Apostles." In *Miracles: Cambridge Studies in their Philosophy and History*, edited by C. F. D. Moule. 165–78. London: Mowbray, 1965.

Lawrence, Roy. "Every Church a Centre of Healing?" *Network* (2001) Issue 46.

Le Fanu, James. *The Rise and Fall of Modern Medicine*. 2nd ed. London: Abacus, 2011.

Bibliography

Levy, L. F. "Epilepsy in Rhodesia, Zambia and Malawi." *African Journal of Medical Science* 1 (1970) 155–60.
Lewis, C. S. *Surprised by Joy: The Shape of My Early Life*. London: Fontana, 1959.
Lewis, D. *Healing: Faith, Fact or Fiction*. London: Hodder & Stoughton, 1989.
Lewis, I. M. *Ecstatic Religion: An Anthropological Study of Spirit Possession and Shamanism*. Harmondsworth, UK: Penguin, 1971.
Lloyd-Jones, D. Martin. *Healing and Medicine*. Eastbourne, UK: Kingsway, 1987.
Lucas, Ernest. *Christian Healing: What Can We Believe?* London: Lynx, 1997.
May, Peter. "Correspondence." *The Church Times* 5 October 1990.
McGrath, Alister E. "Doctrine and Ethics." *Journal of the Evangelical Theological Society* 34 (1991) 145–156.
McLaren, R. *Professions Working Together*. St Marylebone Papers No 8. London: St Marylebone Healing and Counselling Centre. 1992.
MacNutt, Francis. *Healing*. New York: Bantam, 1980.
Mews, S. "The Revival of Spiritual Healing in the Church of England 1920–26." In *The Church and Healing*, edited by W. J. Shiels, 299–331. Oxford: Blackwell, 1982.
Ness, R. C., and R. M. Wintrobe. "The Emotional Impact of Fundamentalist Religious Participation." *American Journal of Orthopsychiatry* 50 (1980) 302–15
Newbiggin, Lesslie. *Foolishness to the Greeks: The Gospel and Western Culture*. Geneva: World Council of Churches, 1986.
Nolen, William. *Healing: A Doctor in Search of a Miracle*. New York: Random House, 1974.
Noll, Richard. *The Jung Cult: Origins of a Charismatic Movement*. Princeton: Princeton University Press, 1994.
Numbers, R .L., and R. C. Sawyer. "Medicine and Christianity in the Modern World." In *Health/Medicine and the Faith Tradition: An Enquiry into Religion and Medicine*, edited by Martin E. Marty, and Kenneth L. Vaux, 153. Philadelphia: Fortress, 1982.
NZPA. "Exorcism Pastor in Court." *The Dominion* (Wellington, NZ) 20 Jan 2001, 3.
Offit, P. A. "Studying Complementary and Alternative Therapies." *Journal of the American Medical Association* 307 (2012) 1803–4.
O'Laoire, S. "An Experimental Study of the Effects of Distant, Intercessory Prayer on Self-esteem, Anxiety, and Depression." *Alternative Therapies in Health and Medicine* 3/6 (1997) 38–53.
Parker, Larry, as told to Don Tanner. *We Let Our Son Die*. Irvine, CA: Harvest House, 1980.
Peters, R. M. "The Effectiveness of Therapeutic Touch: A Meta-analytic Review." *Nursing Science Quarterly* 12 (1) (1999) 52–61.
Peterson, R., and M. Peterson. *Roaring Lion*. Singapore: OMF, 1989.
Pfeifer, S. "Belief in Demons and Exorcism in Psychiatric Patients in Switzerland." *British Journal of Medical Psychology* 67 (1994) 247–58.
Pitcher, George. "The Loony-Tunes Church that Claims to Heal HIV Sufferers Is One of Many Obsessed with Sex and 'Curing' Homosexuals." *Daily Mail* (London) 25 November 2011. Online: http://www.dailymail.co.uk/debate/article-2066123/
Pittler, Max H., and Edzard Ernst. "Complementary Therapies for Neuropathic and Neuralgic Pain: A Systematic Review." *Clinical Journal of Pain* 24 (2008) 731–35.
Powell, L. H., et al. "Religion and Spirituality: Linkages to Physical Health." *American Psychologist* 58/1 (2003) 36–52.
Prince, D. *Expelling Demons*. Fort Lauderdale, FL: Derek Prince Ministries, n.d.

Bibliography

Pytches, D. "New Wine '90." *Church Times* 31 August 1990.
Ramsey, Ian T. *Religious Language: An Empirical Placing of Theological Phrases*. London: SCM, 1957.
Randi, James. *The Faith Healers*. Buffalo, NY: Prometheus, 1978.
———. "The Detection of Fraud and Fakery." *Experientia* 44 (1988) 287–90.
Rose, Louis. *Faith Healing*. Harmondsworth, UK: Penguin, 1971.
Rees, L., and A.Weil. "Integrated Medicine." *British Medical Journal* 322 (2001) 119–20.
Shapiro, Arthur K., and Elaine Shapiro. T*he Powerful Placebo: From Ancient Priest to Modern Physician*. Baltimore: Johns Hopkins University Press, 1997.
Sherman, R., and J. Hickner. "Academic Physicians Use Placebos in Clinical Practice and Believe in the Mind–Body Connection." *Journal of General Internal Medicine* 23/1 (2008) 7–10.
Short, David. "Modern Healing Miracles in Perspective." *Journal of the Christian Medical Fellowship* 33/4 (1987) 26–27.
Sicher, F., et al. "A Randomized Double-blind Study of the Effect of Distant Healing in a Population with Advanced AIDS—Report of a Small Scale Study." *Western Journal of Medicine* 169 (1998) 356–63.
Sims, Andrew. C. P. "Demon Possession: Medical Perspective in a Western Culture." In *Medicine and the Bible*, edited by Bernard Palmer, 165–89. Exeter, UK: Paternoster, 1986.
Singh, Simon, and Edzard Ernst. *Trick or Treatment: The Undeniable Facts about Alternative Medicine*. New York: Norton, 2008.
Skrabanek, Petr. *The Death of Humane Medicine and the Rise of Coercive Healthism*. London: Social Affairs Unit, 1994.
Sloan, Richard P. *Blind Faith: The Unholy Alliance of Religion and Medicine*. New York: St. Martin's, 2006.
——— et al. "Religion, Spirituality and Medicine." *Lancet* 353 (1999) 664–67.
Smart, H. L., et al. "Alternative Medicine Consultations and Remedies in Patients with the Irritable Bowel Syndrome." *Gut* 27 (1986) 826–28.
Smedes, Lewis B. *Ministry and the Miraculous: A Case Study at Fuller Theological Seminary*. Pasadena CA: Fuller Theological Seminary, 1987.
Smith, D. M. "Safety of Faith Healing." *Lancet* i (1986) 621.
So, P. S., et al. "Touch Therapies for Pain Relief in Adults." *Cochrane Database of Systematic Reviews* Issue 4 (Oct 8, 2008) Art. No. CD006535
Spence, C., et al. "The Faith Assembly: A Study of Perinatal and Maternal Mortality." *Indiana Medicine* 77 (1984) 180–83.
———, and T. S. Donaldson. "The Faith Assembly: A Follow-up Study of Faith Healing and Mortality." *Indiana Medicine* 80 (1987) 238–40.
Stewart, James Stuart. *A Faith to Proclaim*. London: Hodder & Stoughton, 1962.
Subritzky, Bill. *Demons Defeated*. Chichester, UK: Sovereign World, 1986.
Thomas, K. J., et al. "Use of Non-orthodox and Conventional Health Care in Great Britain." *British Medical Journal* 302 (1991) 207–10.
Trowell, H. *Study Notes on Faith Healing*. London: Institute of Religion and Medicine, 1969.
Turner, G. "Healing in Church Services." *Journal of the Christian Medical Fellowship* 37/2 (1991) 7–9.
Vermes, Geza. *Providential Accidents: An Autobiography*. New York: Rowan & Littlefield, 1998.

Bibliography

Vincent, C. "Complementary Medicine: State of the Evidence." *Journal of the Royal Society of Medicine* 92 (1999) 170–77.
Wagner, C. Peter, and F. Douglas Pennoyer, editors. *Wrestling with Dark Angels: Toward a Deeper Understanding of the Supernatural Forcs in Spiritual Warfare*. Ventura, CA: Regal, 1990.
Wainwright, Elaine M., editor. *Spirit Possession, Theology, and Identity: A Pacific Exploration*. Hindmarsh, South Australia: ATF Ltd, 2010.
Wampold, B. E., et al. "The Placebo is Powerful: Estimating Placebo Effects in Medicine and Psychotherapy from Randomized Clinical Trials." *Journal of Clinical Psychology* 61 (2005) 835–54.
Whyte, H. A. Maxwell. *Demons and Deliverance*. Springdale, PA: Whitaker House, 1989.
Wilkinson, J. "Healing in Semantics, Creation and Redemption." *Scottish Bulletin of Evangelical Theology* 4 (1986) 17–37.
Wimber, John, and Kevin Springer. *Power Healing*. London: Hodder & Stoughton, 1987.
———. *Power Evangelism*. London: Hodder & Stoughton, 1987.
Wright, F. J. "Healing: An Interpretation of James 5:13–20." *Journal of the Christian Medical Fellowship* 37/1 (1991) 20–21.
Wright, Verna. "A Medical View of Miraculous Healing." In *The Healing Epidemic*, edited by Peter Masters, 202–27. London: Wakeman Trust, 1988.

www.ingramcontent.com/pod-product-compliance
Lightning Source LLC
Chambersburg PA
CBHW032234080426
42735CB00008B/848